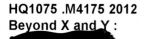

DATE DUE

JAN 1 3 2013	
MAY 1 2 2015	
MAY 1 2 2022	
2/28	

Beyond X and Y

Beyond X and Y

Inside the Science of Gender

Jane McCredie

ROWMAN & LITTLEFIELD PUBLISHERS, INC.
Lanham • Boulder • New York • Toronto • Plymouth, UK

Published by Rowman & Littlefield Publishers, Inc.
A wholly owned subsidary of The Rowman & Littlefield Publishing Group, Inc.
4501 Forbes Boulevard, Suite 200, Lanham, Maryland 20706
www.rowman.com

10 Thornbury Road, Plymouth PL6 7PP, United Kingdom

Copyright © 2011 by Jane McCredie
First Rowman & Littlefield edition published in 2012
Originally published as *Making Girls and Boys: Inside the Science of Sex* in 2011 in
Australia by NewSouth, an imprint of UNSW Press

British Library Cataloguing in Publication Information Available

Library of Congress Cataloging-in-Publication Data

McCredie, Jane.
Beyond X and Y : inside the science of gender / Jane McCredie. -- 1st Rowman Littlefield ed.
p. cm.
Originally published as: Making girls and boys : inside the science of sex / Jane McCredie (Sydney :
University of New South Wales Press, 2011).
Includes bibliographical references and index.
ISBN 978-1-4422-1962-5 (alk. paper)
1. Gender identity. 2. Sex (Psychology) 3. Sex determination, Genetic. I. McCredie, Jane. Making
girls and boys. II. Title.
HQ1075.M4175 2012
305.3--dc23
2012025709

⊗™ The paper used in this publication meets the minimum requirements of American
National Standard for Information Sciences Permanence of Paper for Printed Library
Materials, ANSI/NISO Z39.48-1992.

Printed in the United States of America

For Alice and James

Contents

Preface

When South African athlete Caster Semenya raced away with the women's 800 meters at the athletics world championships in August 2009, it didn't take long for the whispers to start. The eighteen-year-old from an impoverished village of the northern Limpopo looked like a man, people said. Her build, apparent facial hair and the way she moved were all said to demonstrate that she was not a real woman and therefore should not be allowed to compete in female events.

"For me, she is not a woman. She is a man," said Italy's Elisa Cusma Piccione, who ran sixth in the event.

Certainly, the race looked dramatic. Semenya ran with the pack most of the way but around the 600-meter mark began to draw away, leading by 5 meters, then 10, then 15. The footage is surreal, like watching a professional runner compete against a field of amateurs, or an adult outrun a bunch of five-year-olds. Semenya is bigger and taller than her competitors, her powerful build accentuated by the fact that, while all the other women wear briefs, she alone is in lycra shorts. Seen in motion from behind—which of course is how her outraged competitors did see her—you can't help thinking the tight buttocks and muscular thighs do look like those of a man.

In the end, she won by more than 20 meters and an extraordinary margin of 2.5 seconds. Her performance was well short of the world record, but that's not so surprising. The record has remained unchallenged since 1983, back in the days when Eastern European athletes were routinely fed male hormones or similar substances to enhance their strength and endurance. "That world record will never be broken," a veteran sports writer tells me.

In the ensuing media furor, dozens of stories questioned Semenya's female identity. She was said to have had a medal taken away at a primary school athletics competition after complaints that she was really a boy, to have been denied access to female toilets by petrol station attendants, to have engaged in "male" behaviors such as playing football and following world championship wrestling. At the center of the storm was a bewildered teenager, unaccustomed to the glare of publicity, whose most private medical details—including claims she had been found to be a "hermaphrodite"—were apparently leaked to the world's media before she herself had even been made aware of them.

There are many questions you could ask as you watch Semenya fronting the cameras, but most of the discussion was limited to one basic query: "What is she?" South African authorities had apparently relied on a "drop your pants and show us what you've got" approach, but the International Association of Athletics Federations (IAAF) declared the issue to be more complicated than that. Semenya would undergo a range of tests, they announced, with reports to be provided by a gynecologist, endocrinologist (hormone specialist), internal medicine specialist, psychologist, and gender specialist. The different experts would conduct their assessments, contribute their findings and, somehow, from a mess of complex and possibly conflicting information a decision would be reached. It took nearly a year, but the IAAF eventually cleared Semenya to compete in women's events.

Many people were surprised to learn that the question of what makes somebody a man or a woman is not always a straightforward one, but sporting authorities have been grappling with the issue for decades. Concerned that men might fraudulently enter female competition, they have tried various methods of gender verification, from genetic testing to forcing female athletes to parade naked in front of a medical panel. But none of these methods were foolproof because the plain fact is that not everybody fits neatly into one of the two categories of male and female.

For sporting authorities concerned about whether an athlete's biological make-up gives them an advantage over other women, the real question ends up being a much more difficult one: not whether an athlete is female, but whether she is female enough.

Acknowledgments

Many people have contributed to the writing of this book by sharing their life stories, responding to my questions, or sending me information. Some have chosen to remain anonymous so I cannot name them here, but thank them anyway. In particular, I would like to thank:

Aram, Trent Atkinson, Professor Simon Baron-Cohen, Professor Larry Cahill, Carlos Casanova, Craig, James Dando, Associate Professor Peter Eckersall, Delia Falconer, Professor Jennifer Graves, Professor Vincent Harley, Bonnie Hart, Associate Professor Peter Jackson, Karen, Professor Peter Koopman, Liam Leonard, Dr. Linda Mann, Norrie May-Welby, Anna McCredie, Elise McCredie, Ian McCredie, Professor Geoff McFadden, Professor Louise Newman, Professor Harry Ostrer, Peta, David Pledger, Professor Allan Reiss, Professor Lesley Rogers, Associate Professor Darren Russell, Graem Sims, Professor Garry Warne and Professor Jeffrey Zajac.

I thank my original publisher, Stephen Pincock, for his unfailing enthusiasm and support and Phillipa McGuinness for her admirable sang-froid in seeing the book through to publication. Thanks go to everybody at UNSW Press for their talent and commitment and to Marie-Louise Taylor for her sensitive, meticulous editing.

Thank you, too, to the many friends and family members who have maintained interest through the life of this project, especially my parents, Yvonne and David McCredie. The incomparable Guy McEwan has earned my gratitude for his friendship, support, insightful comments on the manuscript and help with the arduous task of transcribing interviews. Most of all, I thank my daughter, Alice McCredie-Dando, for assistance with research and for being the most perceptive reader I have ever met.

Introduction

We know there are two sexes.

Don't we?

Well, yes, we do. More or less.

When a healthy baby is born, the first thing we do is have a look between its legs. If there's a vulva, we declare: "It's a girl!" If there's a penis: "It's a boy!" It's the first label to be applied to us and the first thing anybody asks about a newborn baby. But, as sporting authorities have discovered, even biological sex is not always that simple. And the physical details have nothing on the complex can of worms that is gender identity.

Some feminist and queer theorists have attacked the binary view of male and female as two "opposite" sexes, sometimes even suggesting that not just gender but biological sex itself is a social construct. Because we believe there are two sexes, we are obliged to classify individuals as belonging to one or the other, remaining blind to the ways in which they—we—might not fit the categories.

Caster Semenya, for example, was claimed in some media reports to have a condition called androgen insensitivity syndrome, which sees genetically male babies with testes develop as females because their bodies lack the ability to read male hormones. Although these women have male levels of testosterone, they would not have an advantage over other females in sporting competition because they are unable to use it.

People whose bodies are not clearly one thing or the other are perhaps the most stark example of how inadequate our classifications can be, but to some extent the binary view of sex fails us all. Think about it: there is not a single generalization about males or females that can be applied to every individual

1

member of a particular sex. Women can be tall, hairy, aggressive, or good at map reading. Men may lactate, gossip, stay awake after sex or be good at multitasking.

The theorists' view of anatomical sex as a social construct might seem strange at first glance, but some scientists are also starting to move away from the idea of biology as the fixed basis on which the social artifact of gender is built. Biology and environment are increasingly seen as constantly interacting, constantly affecting each other, to the point where distinctions between biological sex and socially constructed gender become hard to maintain. When our hormone levels fluctuate in response to life events, they change us on a biological level. When we learn new behaviors, when we fall in love, neural connections rewire, changing the actual anatomy of our brains.

All of us—men, women, those who resist easy classification—are products of this dynamic, ever-changing interaction between biology and environment. It begins in the womb and continues until the day we die. So many factors are involved, and the possible interactions between them are so varied and unpredictable, that it becomes almost impossible to make generalizations about the "nature" of human beings or of the two sexes. As a species, we humans are complex, unpredictable, inconsistent, infuriating, and entrancing—we just don't fit into boxes very well.

When it comes to anatomy, we may never know for certain whether Semenya really does belong to the surprisingly large number of people—estimates range from about one in 4500 to as high as one in 50—whose biology does not fit neatly into one of the standard two boxes of male and female. But we do know sporting authorities are not the only ones who find themselves trying to jam non-conformist bodies or minds into nice, clear-cut categories. Governments too have been anxious to ensure that all their citizens fit neatly into either the male or female box, in part at least out of a desire to avoid any possibility of legally sanctioned homosexuality. If you're going to define marriage as being "between one man and one woman," you need to be able to categorize the people involved as clearly one thing or the other—and some regimes go to bizarre lengths to do so. In Iran, where homosexuality can incur the death penalty, the Ayatollah Khomeini himself endorsed a policy that allows (some would say, compels) gay men to have sex-change surgery so that they can become compliant women.

This book had its origins in a case that saw authorities attempting to come to grips with slippery, and many would say confronting, ideas about sex and gender. In 2007, a woman appeared in front of Australia's Family Court seeking permission for her twelve-year-old daughter, code-named Brodie by the court, to become her son. The child wanted to start secondary school as a boy and had threatened self-harm if action was not taken to prevent him going through a female puberty.

Language fails when writing about such a case. So fundamental is sex to our understanding of what constitutes a human being that, in English and most other languages, we are actually incapable of describing somebody without referring to them as either "he" or "she." Brodie, like others who will appear in this book, is somebody whose story cannot easily be contained within such terms. There is no perfect solution to this linguistic dilemma, but I have tried as much as possible to use the language the person or people being described would prefer, albeit with sometimes disconcerting results (the phrases "his clitoris" and "her testes" both appear in this book).

Brodie's story drew a lot of media attention, provoking outrage in some quarters, as cases that challenge our understandings of gender boundaries tend to do. The court's eventual decision that he should be allowed to receive reversible hormone treatment to prevent female puberty was variously described as a tragedy, child abuse, and a failure to address the "real" causes of Brodie's discomfort, seen as lying in the bitterness and anger between his estranged parents and the breakdown of his own relationship with his father, who lived several thousand kilometers away in another state.

In the wake of the case, I wrote an article for a doctors' magazine about gender identity issues in children. Reading the court's judgment was a heart-rending experience. Everybody in this family was in turmoil: from the estranged father, to the anguished mother, to the younger sister, described in the judgment as a "sad little girl." Brodie himself seemed consumed by anger, a rampaging fury that he could not be who he wanted to be, that he was forced to go through the lengthy process of seeking approval for medical treatment. He was "a child in crisis," the family consultant told the court, describing his appearance as that of an angry, intelligent, pre-pubescent boy, dressed in loose, unisex clothing and walking with shoulders hunched and head down.

All the expert witnesses supported the proposed treatment to prevent puberty, agreeing there was a serious risk of self-harm without it. "My understanding is . . . that he sees the idea of going on through life with the spectre of being female, and yet male, so sort of severe a one that he would try and harm himself or undermine his general development," a child psychiatrist told the court.

Brodie's mother too, although she had wavered in her views over whether medical treatment was the right way to go, praying each night that the problem would just go away, was concerned about the risks of doing nothing. She had overheard Brodie crying and yelling on the phone to his father: "I am a boy, Dad, and I will kill myself if I have to live as a girl!"

The father was not represented in court, but he opposed the treatment, believing his daughter was too young to make such a major decision. Although he had said he would support his child no matter what the court decided, the court also heard that he had sent text messages to Brodie, one of which read in part: "I don't believe you can treat me like shit after all I am prepared to do for you . . . I want the little girl up here not some girl who thinks she is a boy . . . You're a nasty little girl [Brodie] with no heart."

In the context of such a volatile family situation, the court and the professionals involved in the case had to work out what they believed would be in the best interest of this troubled child. Suppressing puberty would allow some "breathing time," an endocrinologist told the court, allowing Brodie's anger and the risk of self-harm to subside so that he could address his identity issues in a calmer environment.

The court considered whether those identity issues might just be a phase Brodie was going through.

"[Brodie] convinced me that from the earliest stage of his life he felt male . . . from the very beginning and from my experience with him, he has not wavered in the slightest in his conviction that he always was male and always will be male," the endocrinologist said. Brodie had, he said, a profound and persistent gender identity disorder, "a disorder in which the person is so convinced that they are in fact the other gender that they can't understand why other people don't see them this way."

The psychiatrist agreed: "A tomboy is a girl who has no question about her identity as a girl but just prefers to do masculine things. [Brodie's] core identity is of a male, not of a female wanting to be like a boy." Another psychiatrist had earlier assessed the child as having "a clear, strong and persisting identification with the male gender, which was unchanged since at least the age of four, and seemed irreversible."

Brodie's mother too had seen no signs of change in her child's identity: "From a very early age, [my daughter] identified strongly as a boy and whilst she is a normal female in terms of her anatomy and physiology, I have observed that she really behaves and considers herself to be a boy in every practical sense," she told the court.

After hearing the evidence, the court gave permission for Brodie to receive regular subcutaneous hormonal implants that would suppress ovarian function and estrogen secretion, preventing menstruation and breast development. The initial treatment was fully reversible, but it was expected there would be a later application, perhaps at around age sixteen, to allow administration of the male hormone, testosterone, which would cause non-reversible masculinizing changes such as deepening the voice, growth of the clitoris and muscle development.

Reading the Brodie case, I was overcome by sadness at all this family had had to go through, at the awful dilemma faced by the parents and at the despair and rage endured by the child at the center of it all. But I was also filled with questions. As the mother of a daughter and a son, as a former "tomboy" myself, I had long been fascinated by issues of gender. I had read about and met transsexual adults in the course of my work as a journalist and had occasionally wondered why it was so important to them to change their bodies to fit their sense of self. Why, I had thought, could they not just be the person they were within the body they had? As a young reporter on court rounds, I remembered speaking to a trans woman whose girlfriend had been killed during an assault outside a nightclub and being puzzled that this woman had bothered to change her sex if she was attracted to women anyway (which just goes to show how ignorant I was at age twenty of the complexities of sex, gender and sexual orientation—something we'll come back to later in this book).

Somehow, though, I had never wondered what childhood was like for somebody with what clinicians call persistent gender identity disorder. Perhaps because I had muddled the issues of gender identity and sexuality, I had assumed without really thinking about it that transsexualism would emerge as part of somebody's developing sexual nature—around the time of puberty perhaps, but hardly in toddlerhood. In the course of researching the article for the doctors' magazine, I spoke to psychiatrists, an endocrinologist, a gynecologist and one person, a self-described "transgender lady," who had lived through the experience. All confirmed that a transsexual identity appears early, generally before a child starts school.

The conversations were moving, thought-provoking, enlightening, but they left me confused. If a genetically female child could have an unshakeable conviction from the age of four that he was in fact a boy, what did that tell us about how we all come to inhabit our genders?

I had always tended to think of the sexes as not so much a pair of opposites, but more a spectrum: extreme male at one end, extreme female at the other, and most of us somewhere in between. I once said to a gay friend that I had never wanted to see gender as a straitjacket. "No! More of a frilly pinafore, darling," was his reply. But as I started my research for this book, talking to scientists and to people with radically different relationships to their gender from my own, I began to see even that as an inadequate representation of the full range of human experience.

Biological scientists told me about the various different measures they could use to describe an organism's sex, from chromosomes, to hormones, to reproductive anatomy, to the structure of the brain—not all of which would necessarily line up neatly within the same male or female category. Transsexual people described feeling from early childhood that they were in the "wrong" body, while an intersex woman told me how much she valued the feeling of being outside, of being something more than, the binary.

Increasingly, I found myself thinking that there is not just one, but a series of spectrums. There are chromosomes, the collections of genes that tell our bodies whether we are meant to be male or female or something in between. Then there are the actual bodies we end up with, determined by the interaction between those genes and the hormones that produce our sexual characteristics. There is whatever happens in our brains that helps us to feel like a boy or a girl, to behave like a boy or a girl (whatever that might mean). There is the role we play in society, how those around us see us and what their expectations are of somebody who belongs to the sex we present. And there are other things, too, like our sexual orientation, who we are attracted to and what we like to do with them, that might not be strictly part of our gender identity but seem in some way intertwined with it.

For most of us, all of these spectrums line up in a more or less orderly fashion: chromosomes match our anatomy, our sense of ourselves, and the way we are perceived by others. But there is no necessary relationship between an individual's position on any one spectrum—anatomy, say—and where they sit on any of the others. The myriad intersections of these related, but not identical, scales produce a dizzying array of possible human beings: from the macho straight male to the ultra-feminine lesbian, from the bearded woman to the gay man who started life in a female body.

When I set out to explore the various spectrums of sex, I began with our bodies. I read research into genetics and fetal development, spoke to scientists and doctors, in an attempt to understand how these bodies that are so central to our idea of ourselves as male or female are formed. But other fields of research quickly began to intrude. What could evolutionary theory tell us about how our bodies, and even more intriguingly the brains they carry, have come to be the way they are? Do men and women really have different brains? And, if they do, what does that mean for the psychological development of boys and girls? These are only some of the questions I have found myself trying to answer on a journey through fields of research from evolutionary biology to psychology, from endocrinology to anthropology.

But more of that later. Let's start where it begins for all of us, no matter how many twists and turns we take along the way: with the unpredictable blending of genetic material from two other individuals that encodes, among other things, our sex.

Chapter One

Conceiving Girls and Boys

"What is a man?" I ask endocrinologist Jeffrey Zajac, who has spent many years researching testosterone and the other hormones that help create what we usually think of as maleness.

His response is lengthy, touching on fetal development, intersex conditions, evolution and the ancient Greek idea of perfection, but the answer when it comes is simple: "A male is a sperm-producing organism," he says. "Once you've got the sperm, you don't need the male."

He's right: in one sense that is all a man is, while a woman by the same logic is no more than an egg factory and incubator. At its most basic, the existence of two biologically and genetically distinct sexes is just the mechanism evolution has chosen to allow our and most other animal species to reproduce. Two complementary animals come together, each contributing half of its genetic make-up to create a new individual that is a unique and unpredictable mixture of both parents.

It doesn't have to be this way. Although most hermaphroditic animals can't fertilize themselves, the Central American killifish and some freshwater snails do. Various insects, birds, and reptiles have the ability to overcome a male drought by turning temporarily or permanently to parthenogenesis (literally: virgin birth), a process by which a female produces offspring from her own genetic material without the need for fertilization at all—clones, in effect. Many species of stick insect that follow this procedure have dispensed with males entirely.

Perhaps the biggest advantage of mating, apart from the obvious, lies in its fostering of innovation. As sexless creatures, we would not be switching off the evolutionary process completely—random mutations in our genes could still occur—but we would be hugely reducing the creative diversity that comes from the mingling of two individuals' genes. Still, even some animals that engage in sexual reproduction have a far more flexible approach to it than we humans. Many fish, for example, are capable of being either male or female, depending on environmental conditions and the availability of partners. For some species, changing sex is part of the natural life cycle, in a process known as sequential hermaphroditism.

The animated film *Finding Nemo* would have told a different story if it had portrayed the life of its clownfish heroes more accurately. All of these cheerfully colored reef fish start their lives as pre-pubescent males so the protagonist, Nemo, was correctly cast as a young boy. But his widowed father Marlin, who undertakes the heroic journey from tropical Queensland to Sydney Harbor to rescue his abducted son, is an impossible creature. Marlin's bereavement would in fact have triggered a quite different journey, one that saw him transform himself into a female, the ultimate achievement of a clownfish's existence. Clownfish live in small colonies, consisting of one breeding pair and up to four pre-pubescent males who must wait their turn to move up in the hierarchy. The largest male in any group becomes female, while the next largest is the reproductive male. When the female dies, that leading male then takes her place while the next largest male steps into the paternal role, and so on.

The process can go in the other direction. Another tropical fish, the bluestreak cleaner wrasse, is the beautician (or perhaps the carwash attendant) of the coral reef. These small, brightly colored fish congregate in locations called cleaning stations where they feed off the parasites and dead tissue on bigger fish that come there to be serviced. The largest adult in a group of wrasse is a territorial male and, when he dies, the biggest female will change sex to take his place. This sexual mutability is an efficient reproductive strategy, allowing the fish to maximize their chances of passing on their genes even when circumstances change around them.

THE GREAT EGG AND SPERM RACE

Q: Why does it take 150 million sperm to fertilize one egg?
A: Because none of them will ask for directions.

A joke that plays on one of the stereotypes about men also raises a serious question: why does it take so many sperm to fertilize a single egg? Nature generally abhors waste. The death of one living entity provides food for another. The parasites on one animal are eaten by another that, like the bluestreak cleaner wrasse, grooms the host, thus improving its health and resistance to disease. So why use physical resources to produce millions of wasted sperm? Wouldn't males be better off investing in a single high-quality sperm, as females do in a single egg?

The classic answer is that the frantic race up the birth canal is an example of Darwinian survival of the fittest, a race to the death in which the fittest and most agile sperm (or perhaps the sperm with the best sense of direction) wins, ensuring the best possible genetic material is transmitted to the resulting fetus. But still, 150 million? Wouldn't it be just as effective and use fewer resources if we had, say, one hundred sperm in the race? Many have sought some kind of metaphor for maleness and femaleness in the differences between sperm and egg. In fact, the story of conception can often sound a bit like Sleeping Beauty, with the courageous hero making a perilous journey through hostile territory to awaken the unconscious princess. Writing at the end of the nineteenth century, zoologist Patrick Geddes drew a clear link between the personalities of the germ cells and those of their owners: the small and active sperm belonged to the smarter, more independent, more energetic sex, while the sluggish, well-fed egg was the product of the more patient and intuitive one.

Still today, many theories about the "natural" mating and relational behavior of men and women rest on the enormous numerical imbalance between their germ cells. Because sperm are cheap, males are said to be impelled to spread them as far and wide as possible, with little thought for the quality or even the survival of any resulting offspring. Female mammals, on the other hand, have a far smaller number of eggs and make a much greater investment in development of the embryo and infant, leading them to be much choosier about prospective mates (we'll come back to these ideas in the next chapter).

I can't help wondering why, if competition is essential for quality assurance in sperm, the same doesn't apply to eggs. Wouldn't it make sense for women to produce a few dozen eggs each month that could race each other down the Fallopian tubes to prove their fitness by being first to reach the incoming tide of spermatozoa? And, in fact, as I read more about the process of conception, I start to get a glimmering that the egg waiting in the Fallopian tube has already won its own Darwinian struggle.

Unlike males, who manufacture new sperm constantly from puberty into old age at a rate of about four million per hour, females form all their germ cells while they are still in the womb. Halfway through gestation, the baby girl's developing ovaries contain perhaps seven million cells with the potential to become eggs. By the time she reaches puberty, a vicious weeding out process has seen these reduced to perhaps 200 thousand, a pool from which between twelve and thirty eggs are selected each month to see which can ripen most quickly. The egg that out-muscles its competitors is the one that gets released into the Fallopian tube to meet, if it is lucky, an approaching sperm.

The story of conception, of that great sperm race toward the waiting egg, may be familiar to us now, but it is a relatively recent discovery. Although humans would no doubt have discovered the link between the sexual act and pregnancy early in their history—from the simple fact that no virgin ever conceived—the mechanics of how this worked were a closed book.

The ancient Greeks formulated a number of theories, most of them based around various fluids. Pythagoras thought male semen gave rise to the noble parts of the fetus, while "female semen" gave rise to the gross parts. Hippocrates believed each parent contributed a liquor containing a vital principle or seed. If the seed of both parents was strong, the child would be a boy. If weak, the child would be a girl. Aristotle argued an egg was created by the mingling of semen and menstrual blood, with the father contributing the spirit or soul to the new child. The sex of the child was determined by the weather in the uterus: hot and dry meant a boy, cold and damp a girl.

The third-century Talmudic thinker, Rabbi Simlai, based his theories on the difference in color between menstrual blood and semen. The mother, he suggested, must provide the dark elements of the fetus: the skin, flesh, blood, hair, and dark parts of the eye. The father would contribute the bones, tendons, nails and the white of the eye.

Modern understandings of human reproduction have their origins in the seventeenth and eighteenth centuries. The existence of an egg in mammals was first suggested in 1651 by William Harvey, the English scientist best known for first describing the circulation of the blood, though it would be nearly two centuries before the egg's existence was confirmed by observation. Sperm first came into view in 1678, when Dutchman Anton van Leeuwenhoek reported seeing millions of little animalcules in fish, frog and mammal semen examined under a microscope he had built himself.

It was still not understood how these tiny wriggling things and the hypothetical egg might combine to create offspring, however. Many early scientists took a "preformationist" view, believing God had created the homunculus, or tiny preformed fetus, in complete form inside the egg (or, as some believed, the sperm), with its only task being to grow to full size within the mother's womb. Of course, if you were present in complete form inside your mother's egg, then she too must have been inside her own mother's egg, and so on through an endless series of Russian dolls all the way back to the original creation. The eighteenth-century Swiss preformationist, Albrecht von Haller, went so far as to calculate the number of complete human beings God must have nested within Eve's ovaries on the sixth day of creation. Based on the Earth's age, which Biblical sources put at five thousand to six thousand years, he determined this to be at least 200 billion individual souls.

The Estonian-born embryologist, Karl von Baer, is generally credited with discovering the mammalian egg and its source in the ovary when he dissected ovarian follicles and inspected their contents in 1827:

Led by curiosity . . . I opened one of the follicles and took up the minute object on the point of my knife, finding that I could see it very distinctly and that it was surrounded by mucus. When I placed it under the microscope I was utterly astonished, for I saw an ovule just as I had already seen them in the tubes, and so clearly that a blind man could hardly deny it.

By the end of the nineteenth century, scientists had described the entry of sperm into the mammalian egg and had begun to understand the early development of the embryo. But an even more important discovery was still to come: that of the chromosomes and the genes that cluster in them.

GENES MAKETH THE MAN

I ring my father, a medical specialist and amateur mathematician, with a question. Is it possible to calculate how many ways there are for the genomes of two humans to be combined? Or, in other words, how many distinct individuals would one couple be theoretically capable of producing?

"Oh," he says, uncharacteristically flummoxed. "But that would be on the scale of the number of stars in the universe or drops of water in the ocean. Even the most powerful computer couldn't calculate it."

Predictably enough, though, he rings me back a few hours later, having put down his cryptic crossword to give it a shot.

"Seventy trillion," he says.

Who knows how close that estimate is, but we do know the number of possible variations is huge. Yet each of these potential humans would be remarkably similar too, sharing physical traits that have remained largely unchanged since modern humans first emerged on the African savannah a few hundred thousand years ago. Encoded in our genome is the manual for our development in utero, the genes that tell cells how to group together and form a heart, a kidney, or a liver. There are genes for eye, hair, and skin color, for susceptibility to disease, for intelligence, perhaps even for various personality types. While we still don't know what all our genes do—and some of them appear to do nothing at all, remnants perhaps of some long-vanished genetic pattern in slime or another of our most distant ancestors—we do know that we carry two copies of each of them, one from the egg and one from the sperm, though usually only one of these will be active. The other is there as a kind of insurance policy, allowing errors to be corrected. It can also be passed on to our descendants even though it has not been active in us, which is how we sometimes see traits skip a generation.

Because they are designed to combine with each other, the sperm and egg carry a single copy of each gene, organized into twenty-three chromosomes, half the number found in any other cell in the body. They are in effect half cells, created by the splitting in two of a primordial germ cell, in a process called meiosis. The primordial cell starts out the same in the two sexes—whether it produces sperm or eggs will depend entirely on whether it finds itself inside a testis or not—but there is a key difference between the sexes when it comes to meiosis.

The reason every sperm and egg carries a unique genetic recipe is that, during meiosis, the forty-six chromosomes in the primordial germ cell line up in pairs and swap matched genetic material more or less randomly from one side to the other. This is how a paternal grandfather's gene for blue eyes can end up in the same sperm as a maternal grandmother's snub nose. In female meiosis, when two eggs are created from the primordial cell, this lining up process is relatively straightforward as all the chromosomes match, including the two X chromosomes found in genetic females. Males, however, carry one X chromosome, inherited from their mother, and a Y chromosome, inherited from their father, which means each of their primordial germ cells will produce one male and one female sperm. This is why it is the father's sperm that determines the sex of the future embryo.

Sex doesn't have to be determined genetically in this way. In some animals, such as turtles and crocodiles, the environment plays the primary role in determining sex of offspring, with ambient temperatures while the eggs are being incubated determining whether babies will hatch male or female. But the mammalian genetic method tends to be described as representing evolutionary "progress" because it makes our sex ratios more stable. Imagine if global warming led to our producing only boy babies, or if people living in polar regions could produce only girls. It can, though, be argued that the alternative method also has its evolutionary advantages precisely because it is more responsive to changing environmental conditions.

Researchers have long sought evidence that the sex ratio in humans also varies with changes in external circumstances but, despite a small increase in births of males after both world wars, clear proof has been hard to come by. Women too have tried to influence the sex selection of their babies by inserting various substances into their vaginas or timing sexual contact for a particular stage of their menstrual cycle, though again there is no evidence such maneuvers have a higher success rate than leaving it to chance.

Although men and women appear quite different anatomically, the two sexes actually share the vast majority of their thirty thousand or so genes, all but the forty-five of them that live on that diminutive Y chromosome, which are the exclusive property of males. For most of human history, the existence of the sex-determining X and Y chromosomes remained unsuspected. People assumed the sex of babies resulted, in a more reptilian fashion, from conditions within the womb as they developed. This led to women being congratulated and rewarded if they were prolific producers of sons. But it could also lead to those who managed to produce only daughters being shunned or, as in the case of some of King Henry VIII of England's unfortunate wives, executed.

As we now know, it was Henry's sperm rather than his wives' eggs that were responsible for his female offspring, though that too is a quite recent discovery. Even after the sex chromosomes were first identified at the start of the twentieth century, it took another fifty years for science to appreciate that the Y chromosome was the one that determined sex. Early researchers had assumed it was the presence of the second X chromosome in females that was the determining factor. Once again, there is no necessary reason why it has to be this way. In birds, it is the female who carries both sex chromosomes and thus determines the sex of offspring.

Because they have both X and Y chromosomes, men have all the genes required for female development, which goes some way toward explaining why it is so easy for things to go off course during the complex process of achieving biological maleness. It may play no role in sex determination in humans but, like the egg, the X chromosome is a much bigger and more robust creature than its male counterpart, containing about a thousand genes compared with the Y's meager forty-five. Geneticist Jennifer Graves, who has done extensive research into the evolution of the sex chromosomes, describes the X as the "smart and sexy" chromosome because so many of its genes relate to male reproductive health or to intelligence, in some cases both within the same gene. (Graves is rather less flattering about the Y chromosome as we'll see.)

The reasons for this "brains and balls" coincidence, as Graves puts it, have caused considerable debate in scientific circles. Unlikely as it may seem, the X is actually a good home for genes that give males a reproductive advantage. Because males have only one copy of the chromosome, genes that enhance testis or sperm development will always be expressed if they are housed there, whereas in any of the autosomal (non-sex) chromosomes they would have to battle it out with a second, possibly less advantageous, version of the gene. It is harder to pin down the reasons behind the clustering of genes related to intelligence though it is possible this might also relate to male reproductive advantage, given that brains might make somebody a more attractive mating prospect.

The very quality that makes the female chromosome a good home for genes that provide a male reproductive advantage also, however, makes men more vulnerable to mutations in any of the genes the X carries. Because they only have one copy of these genes, men will always feel the impact of a defective gene on the X, whereas women have a second copy to fall back on. This is why X-linked conditions such as haemophilia and red-green color blindness are so much more common in men than in women.

The Y chromosome, of course, cannot carry genes that are needed by both sexes and much of its genetic material consists in repetitive sequences with no apparent function. But it does carry one very important gene that came to our attention about twenty years ago.

In the late 1980s, researchers around the world were on the hunt for the genetic origins of maleness, the single gene somewhere on the Y chromosome that was assumed to divert the embryo from the female path. One of those researchers was Peter Koopman, a young Australian geneticist working in Robin Lovell-Badge's Medical Research Council Laboratory in London. Koopman and I had been friends as teenagers, when he was a poetry-writing science student and I was neglecting my studies in prehistoric archaeology and English literature. Over intervening decades, we had mostly lost touch until a late autumn day when I went to see him at the lab he now runs as a professor at the University of Queensland.

When researchers began their hunt for the male gene, one of their investigative paths was to look at the genomes of a small group of intersex people: those with two X chromosomes, chromosomal females who had developed as anatomically typical, though infertile, males. The hypothesis, which proved to be correct, was that a gene that was normally found on the Y chromosome would be found to have been accidentally transferred onto a paternal X chromosome during meiosis. (XX males are infertile because, although they have the primary male gene, they lack several other genes involved in sperm creation that also live on the Y chromosome.)

Once a potential gene had been identified in these intersex people, the next step was to test its effects. To do this, the Lovell-Badge team set about literally turning a female mouse embryo into a male. The team removed a fertilized egg with XX chromosomes from a pregnant mouse and injected it with the candidate gene—which would come to be known as *Sry*, or sex-determining region Y—before reimplanting the egg into a foster mother. Keenly aware that they were not the only ones looking for the gene, they rushed into the experiment without all the painstaking preparatory work that would normally be part of creating a transgenic animal.

"We were really lucky," Koopman remembers. "In most cases, if you're making a transgene, you splice together bits of two different genes, one of which ensures that the gene's going to be active when you want it to be, like the on/off switch on a breadmaker, and the other that makes the protein that does what you want it to do, like the breadmaker itself. Usually, you've got time to figure out what two bits to put together to make the thing work. But when we discovered *Sry* we didn't know which part was which. So, we just had to take a big chunk of DNA that we knew had *Sry* in it, inject it into mouse eggs and hope for the best. The chances of the experiment working were miniscule."

"But, amazingly," he says with a laugh, "the gene was active at the right time and place and the experiment worked. And the rest is history."

What he means when he says the experiment worked is that the injection of the gene turned an XX mouse embryo into a male, albeit an infertile one with smaller than normal testes. This extraordinary experiment proved that a single gene could under the right circumstances trigger a male developmental path in a chromosomal female.

Koopman may be a proud parent but he is under no illusions about the gene he helped discover. *Sry* is a pretty pathetic creature, he says, and the reason for this is its home on the Y chromosome.

"Normally, every cell has got two copies of every chromosome," he explains. "And if a gene on one copy of chromosome 7 develops a problem—some sort of mutation—there are correctional methods where enzymes recognise a defect and fix it up by reading from the second copy. But the Y chromosome doesn't have a second copy—it's on its own. If a problem develops in a gene on the Y chromosome, there's no correctional mechanism. And so its genes are literally falling apart."

"*Sry*—the gene on which all sex differences rest—just limps along only barely able to function."

It's lucky for men, and the survival of our species, that so many other male genes reside on the X chromosome or elsewhere in the genome where they can be checked for errors.

Graves, with her evolutionary perspective, has charted the Y chromosome's decline over hundreds of millions of years and believes its days are numbered. Many of its genes have disappeared altogether over that time, leaving it an impoverished remnant of what it might once have been, while others no longer perform any useful function that we can discern. The decrepit creature that remains is, says Graves, best categorized as a "selfish wimp."

"This degraded Y chromosome is a wimp by any measure," she writes. "[It] is disappearing fast, and, indeed, its future looks grim."

Several species of rodent have, in fact, already dispensed with the Y in favor of sex-determining genes elsewhere on the genome. The pace of evolution is slow, however, so the human Y is safe for some time to come. Based on the rate of gene loss from the chromosome over the last 300 million years or so, Graves predicts its eventual demise in humans to be about fourteen million years in the future. We can only speculate about what might replace the chromosome at that point. The death of the Y might spell the end of us as a species, or it might usher in a burst of new hominid species with an entirely different way of determining sex, or even a different means of reproduction—parthenogenesis perhaps.

THE WAR OF THE SEXES

Six weeks after conception, the human embryo floats in a dark, liquid world, its speck of a heart beating at a frantic pace. Not much bigger than a cashew nut and curled in on itself, it looks vaguely reptilian with its primitive limb buds and spine curving round into a tail. Only the huge, misshapen head speaks of its human future.

This early in development, there are no visible differences between the female and male embryo. Anatomically, it has everything it needs to become either a girl or a boy. Internally, its future gonads (ovaries or testes) form two genital ridges, bulges of tissue near the back of the abdominal cavity. Primordial germ cells—the future egg or sperm—have already begun to congregate here, after forming outside the embryo on the lining of the yolk sac and migrating through the embryonic gut, proliferating along the way.

Two sets of sex ducts have also begun to develop, one male, one female. The female Müllerian ducts will, if they are allowed to survive, eventually turn into Fallopian tubes, the uterus and the upper part of the vagina. The male Wolffian ducts will, again if they survive, form the ducts that conduct sperm from the testes to the penis. The expert on reproductive biology, R. H. F. Hunter, has suggested the presence of both male and female duct systems could be a hangover from our evolutionary past, harking back to reptilian days when environmental factors rather than genes determined the developing embryo's sex.

Externally, the tiny human embryo has the beginnings of a phallus, the genital tubercle that will eventually transform into either a clitoris or a penis. Paired urogenital folds will become either a female's labia minora or the flesh enclosing the penile urethra. Outside them, the labioscrotal swelling will either fuse to form the scrotum or remain separate as the labia majora.

The reproductive organs are the only ones in our bodies that have this bipotentiality, or capacity to take two very different developmental paths. You don't see kidneys suddenly doing an about-turn and transforming themselves into hearts. After six weeks, though, the embryo is on the verge of ending its sexually indifferent phase. Over the weeks that follow, it will begin to develop distinctly female organs—unless, that is, the activation of that single gene on the Y chromosome sets off the cascade of male development.

It seems the Bible got it wrong. Far from creating woman as an afterthought to be a companion to man, nature devised the female sex first, with the male a relative newcomer in evolutionary terms. The first animals probably reproduced by parthenogenesis, or some other asexual means, until some aberrant females began mutating to develop the physical characteristics we associate with males, and the two sexes were born. Or so the conventional scientific account of mammalian development would have it: the female, it is often said, is the "default," the sex that will develop in the absence of a specific intervention to create maleness.

As we've seen, that intervention in humans is initiated by a gene on the Y chromosome called *SRY*. (Scientific convention has it that the mouse gene is called *Sry*, while the human gene is capitalized: *SRY*.) The male embryo largely ignores this substance until, at the end of the sixth week after conception, the gene springs into action in the supporting cells of the genital ridge. Actually, given *SRY*'s feebleness, it might be more accurate to say the gene falters into action but, fortunately, it has henchmen to draw upon. It quickly activates other more robust male genes elsewhere in the genome that do much of its work for it.

Under the influence of *SRY*, the supporting cells in what will become the testis turn into Sertoli cells whose role is to protect and nourish future sperm. Without the male gene, these same entities would become the granulosa cells that perform a similar function in the ovary. However, the weakness of the *SRY* gene makes this anything but a straightforward process. The gene may not activate in all cells of the developing gonad, or it may activate at too low a dose or too late in the process to preempt female development. Geneticist Peter Koopman describes it as a war between two opposing pathways waged on a molecular level:

> There are some cells trying to make female gonads, and other cells trying to make male gonads, so there's a bit of a battle going on there. Even within the same cell, it seems that these two pathways are actively trying to compete with each other.

Often, it's a case of "whoever shouts loudest wins," says Koopman, which leaves *SRY* at a disadvantage given its feeble voice. Left unchecked, the battle could see the chromosomally male embryo develop an ovotestis, a gonad containing testicular tubules surrounded by external ovarian structures. Fortunately for males, the Sertoli cells have developed tactics to compensate for their creator's genetic weakness, using a combination of peer pressure and molecular hit squads to eliminate their female competition. The cells secrete two molecules, one that encourages reluctant companions to follow them down the male path even when *SRY* has failed to activate, the other that recognizes developing granulosa cells and, as Koopman puts it, "bumps them off":

> These are mechanisms that don't have to occur in any other developing tissues where embryonic cells can only continue to mature or else stop developing and die. But the gonad's really interesting and unique—and this is what I've spent a lot of my time studying—in that there's two options for how it can mature. The same cell type has the option of becoming either Sertoli cells, a cell type

normally found in a testis, or granulosa cells, which are normally found in the
ovary. If one of these options is blocked, the cell doesn't simply stop developing but instead starts to follow the other route. So, in a developing gonad, it's
important to have all these cells following the same program.

Once the Sertoli cells have differentiated, they give out chemical signals that
prompt the germ cells to start the process of becoming sperm. Cords containing both germ and Sertoli cells begin to develop that will eventually become
the seminiferous tubules of the testis. And between the cords emerges a new
type of cell that will, more than anything else, guide the rest of the embryo's
development as a male.

These are the Leydig cells and their role is to produce the hormone many
see as the essence of maleness: testosterone. This testosterone is converted
into a derivative, dihydrotestosterone, that guides the development of the
male reproductive system, stimulating the genital tubercle to lengthen into a
penis, the urogenital folds to merge into the underside of the shaft, the labioscrotal swellings to fuse as the scrotum and the Wolffian ducts to develop.

Many scientists also believe testosterone produced by the fetal testes
helps to structure the brain of the growing fetus, establishing the neurological
framework for a future male gender identity. The function of a second surge
of testosterone in boys immediately after birth, which sees their levels of the
hormone briefly match those of an adult male, has yet to be explained, but
some believe it too might play a role in brain development. (We do know that
it is why newborn boys so often surprise their carers by having erections.)
Some scientists believe this early influence of testosterone actually creates a
"male brain," a concept we will come back to in chapter 4. The female brain,
in this view, is seen as the "default" position, the organ that forms in the
absence of testosterone, in much the same way as the female anatomy is seen
as the default.

Testosterone is not the only hormone produced in the fetal testes. The
Sertoli cells produce a hormone of their own, anti-Müllerian hormone
(AMH), which causes the female duct system to wither, leaving only vesti-
gial remnants attached to the testis and prostate.

While all this is happening in the male embryo, the female is following
her own developmental path, albeit one that is initiated a few weeks later
than in the male. If *SRY* does not activate during that crucial window around
the end of the embryo's sixth week, female development begins, with the
formation of cords in the outer region of the primitive gonad, the cortex.
Unlike the testis, which will still form in the absence of germ cells (though it
will never produce sperm), the ovary requires germ cells to develop. These
cells congregate in the cortex, while the medulla or inner region of the gonad
begins to degenerate, just as the cortex has degenerated in the male. Within
the growing fetus, the surviving germ cells enter meiosis, splitting into two

cells, each with half the normal number of chromosomes. These developing eggs are then surrounded by a layer of granulosa cells that will eventually become the ovarian follicles.

In the absence of testosterone, female genitals develop and the Wolffian ducts degenerate. With no AMH to suppress them, the Müllerian ducts begin their transformation into the internal female organs.

The description of female development as a "default" is sometimes criticized as implying simply passivity or absence, although scientists stress it does not mean the female path is any less active than the male. The primordial gonad in both sexes is just a tiny speck of tissue that has to develop very quickly into a complex structure, including many different cell types that communicate with each other and are organized in the right spatial arrangement. This probably requires the involvement of dozens, if not hundreds, of genes in both sexes, many of which remain to be identified or to have their roles fully explained. The key difference is that the female process kicks in slightly later in development, allowing a brief window for *SRY* to take action. The view of the female as the default has perhaps led to it being less studied than the male, however, and it is certainly less well understood, as Hunter writes:

> Maleness tends to be given special prominence in discussions of mammalian sexual differentiation, with femaleness being treated essentially as the permissive, secondary or alternative condition (i.e. the default pathway) in the absence of the prior action of any male-determining sequences. Perhaps this general interpretation should be open to modification . . . and rather more active consideration given to the positive steps involved in the formation of an ovary—which itself should be viewed as a specific and incisive process stemming from appropriate gene-regulated events, even though occurring slightly later than the male gonadal pathway.

Perhaps it's not surprising, given that we all start out with the potential to become either male or female, that things can sometimes take an unexpected turn. Embryos with XY chromosomes are particularly vulnerable because that inner female is just waiting behind the thin veneer of maleness for an opportunity to emerge. The achievement of biological maleness requires a whole cascade of events to take place: *SRY* and its subordinate genes must activate properly, the Sertoli cells must fulfill their policeman role, the testis must produce the necessary hormones, and the body must be able to read them. And, when it comes to sexual differentiation, timing is everything, as Koopman explains:

> If you slow down the developmental pathway involved in lung development, you'll probably still end up with a lung, just probably a small one. But, if the signals for male sexual development are delayed for some reason, the embryo

seems to think that those signals are never going to come and so it starts to get on with the job of developing as a female. There's very little spare time in sexual development, and the embryo can't wait around.

Chapter Two

The Evolving Man and Woman

The first thing that strikes me when I start looking into evolutionary biology, and the more recent research field of evolutionary psychology, is that these guys are *obsessed* with sex.

Who would have thought you could construct a theory of human sexuality based on the relative sizes of primate testicles? Or the rather unpleasant mating habits of the elephant seal? For many who take the evolutionary perspective, sexuality, and just about any other human behavior, can be explained by looking at how the brains of the earliest humans—or even our more distant animal ancestors—might have evolved to meet the demands of their environment. Look hard enough and you'll find an evolutionary rationale for everything from boys' liking for rough-and-tumble play to women's supposed greater verbal fluency.

The problem for modern humans is that the environment we supposedly evolved to fit is not our own complex, digitized world but that of our hunter-gatherer ancestors, who lived on the African savannah a couple of hundred thousand years ago. We are as a result fundamentally at odds with our evolved selves, or so the theory goes.

When it comes to looking at the two sexes, and evolutionary psychologists spend a lot of time doing just that, the approach tends to lead to a view of men and women as utterly, irreconcilably different from each other. Inside every anxious male bank worker on the morning commuter train is a primal hunter, whose instincts would have him ranging the land in all his physical splendor scanning the forests for prey, while the marketing executive toting her briefcase beside him is really designed to be back in her cave raising her children communally and making everything agreeable for his triumphant return. If you believe some of the more ludicrous popular texts spouting such views—and millions of readers around the world apparently do—much of the modern malaise, and just about all the difficulties in relationships between men and women, can be ascribed to our denial of such hard-wired imperatives inherited from our most distant ancestors.

Although there's no doubt our brains would have been as subject to the forces of evolution as any other part of us, perhaps more so given their capacity to enhance our prospects of survival when we use them well, there are a couple of problems with such views. One is the assumption that we ourselves have not changed since the long ago days of the Pleistocene; the other is that we don't really know very much about how our earliest ancestors lived, how they divided up the various tasks that had to be accomplished in the course of the day, or how they related to each other in their more intimate moments.

Biological anthropologist James Holland Jones, from Stanford University, writes that, although he believes the complex organ of the brain must have been created by evolutionary selection, he does not believe that many of the claims currently made for evolutionary psychology resist detailed scrutiny:

> I happen to think that the whole sex-differences in sexual preferences thing is the most overplayed finding in all of evolutionary science. In class, I refer to this work as Men-Are-From-Mars Evolutionary Psychology. The basic idea is to take whatever tired sexual stereotype that you'd hear in a second rate stand-up comedian's monologue, or read about in airport bookstore self-help tracts and dress it up as the scientifically proven patrimony of our evolutionary past. Ugh.

The claims of some evolutionary psychologists can indeed seem highly speculative, more intriguing philosophical inquiry than scientific method. Part of the problem is that the theorists have no option but to start with contemporary behavior and then work backward in the hunt for an evolutionary imperative that might underlie it. It's interesting, often thought-provoking, but I can't imagine how you could ever *prove* any of it.

Because we know so little about actual Pleistocene society, many of the claims made about the social organization of our most remote ancestors are based on observation of either our primate relatives or contemporary hunter-gatherer societies, such as the !Kung of southern Africa or Australian Aboriginal people. So, for example, because male chimpanzees have been observed giving females meat when mating with them, it is suggested the earliest men swapped meat for sex, establishing an evolutionary framework that helps explain the male breadwinner of the 1950s (never mind that this has not been the pattern in most human societies before or since).

Such claims tend to assume evolution magically stopped at the end of the Pleistocene, when humans first began to abandon nomadic lifestyles for farming about ten thousand years ago. Although it's true ten thousand years is not long in evolutionary terms, there is in fact plenty of evidence that we have continued to evolve as a species since then, and some of our adaptations have occurred specifically in response to changes in our way of life, as we'll see later in this chapter. It also seems fallacious to assume either chimpanzees or modern hunter-gatherers somehow represent the ancestors of today's humans: they too could be expected to have changed, both genetically and culturally, since the Pleistocene (or, in the case of the chimps, about five million years ago, since that is when our evolutionary paths diverged).

Even more problematic is that we still don't really understand the contribution genetics makes to our behavior and, so complex are the interactions between genes and environment, maybe we never will. Learned behaviors can also be passed on through generations even in our primate cousins, making it difficult to distinguish them from those that may be encoded in the genes. Behaviors that seem to us so intrinsic to our nature as humans that they must surely be hard-wired could just as easily have originated in some distant past and been passed on from parent to child over the generations since, without any genetic underpinning at all.

Perhaps it's not surprising that we seek to understand the present by looking so far into the past. Since scientists early last century first identified the tiny hereditary molecules that live within each cell of our body, we have come to think of our genes as an irresistible force, a road map for our lives that we are more or less powerless to resist. Charles Darwin may not have known about genes when he came up with his theory of evolution, but the two concepts have been more or less seamlessly blended together since. Genes are the substances through which evolution acts, with those that enhance reproductive success more likely to be passed on from one generation to the next. Genes that promote health, survival, fertility and attractiveness to potential sexual partners have an obvious evolutionary advantage over those that predispose us to disease, premature mortality, infertility or unattractiveness.

If all human beings shared the same environment and the same challenges, they would be likely to evolve in similar ways, always allowing for the role of chance mutations. But, in fact, it's obvious that humans in different parts of the globe have evolved in different ways to suit their particular environments. Northern Europeans, for example, evolved paler skins to allow them to synthesize more vitamin D from scarce sunlight, thus improving their bone and general health and making reproductive success more likely. But, because evolution is usually a very slow process, those Europeans' descendants who later migrated to hotter parts of the world, like Australia, have not yet had time to evolve back to the darker skins that would protect them from their new home's harsher sun. And, if you're hoping we'll evolve to meet the challenges of climate change, be warned that we could be facing the next ice age before our genes catch up.

What does all this mean for men and women? The one indisputable distinction between the two sexes is that they play different roles in reproduction—and this is considered to be the driver of their divergent evolutionary paths. Because female animals almost always make a greater biological investment in their offspring, evolutionary theory would suggest this should encourage them to adopt a more conservative mating strategy, seeking fewer but higher quality partners, while males compete with each other for access to the largest possible number of partners regardless of quality. This is the classic explanation for the wide range of mating displays male animals perform in an attempt to convince reluctant females they offer better genetic material than their competitors.

The fact that males *can* just deposit their sperm and move on, paying no more mind to any possible offspring that will result from the donation, is often extrapolated into a view that this constitutes the *natural* behavior of the male animal. This natural behavior is, in humans, only reined in by the myriad social constraints we have placed around the process of reproduction. Men, or so the argument goes, are destined by nature to spread their seed as far and wide as possible, focusing on producing the greatest possible quantity of offspring with little regard for quality. Women, on the other hand, must make a far greater investment in each child and are capable of producing a far smaller number over the course of a lifetime. So, women it is said are forced to focus on quality, trying to choose the best possible genetic material in the male they mate with.

It sounds plausible enough, but nature itself throws up quite a few challenges to this "natural" view. Humans are not the only animal species in which the males make a considerable investment in their offspring. In many bird species, for example, partners mate for life. While the female makes a slightly greater investment, to the extent that she nourishes the developing egg within her body initially, both parents take responsibility for sitting on the egg to keep it warm after it is laid and for feeding and training the chicks after they hatch.

It is clear that male animals can adopt more than one strategy to maximize their chances of perpetuating their genes. They *can* go for quantity, as the herding animals generally do, but they can also go for quality, committing themselves to playing an ongoing role in the nurture of their offspring as do the birds and some mammals such as the prairie voles. Both sexes can, and perhaps do in many species, adopt a mixed strategy, where they choose one lifelong partner to share the work of raising young but also take any opportunities that come along to access particularly high-quality genetic material through a casual encounter.

It seems to me there are good evolutionary reasons why the "scatter your seed far and wide" approach might not in fact be the most successful one for human males. The human infant is unusually helpless and remains in a state of dependence for a length of time that is unparalleled among animals. The reason for this lies in the complexity of our brains and social structures: a prolonged childhood is necessary because we have so much to learn before we can become fully functioning members of society. As a result, human young require considerable investment from both parents if they are to be given the best chance of survival. Whether that investment takes the form of nurturing, teaching the skills needed for adulthood, or providing food and other basic needs, it is likely to be substantial for both mother and father, meaning their evolutionary imperatives could actually be quite similar. A father who is going to devote substantial resources to one woman and her offspring is likely to be just as concerned about her genetic fitness as she is about his, which is perhaps why we see mating display behaviors in both human sexes whereas in most animals these are restricted to the males.

In the animal world generally, females usually choose their sexual part-ners from an ever-willing throng of males, who are forced to compete in whatever way they can for attention. Strategies range from the completely impractical peacock's tail, to elaborate dances, house building, or gifts de-signed to show the male will be a good provider for his children. Australian bower birds, for example, build an elaborate structure out of grass and twigs and decorate it with all the bright blue objects they can find. I've often thought it must have been a frustrating life for the male birds before the advent of plastic because there's not a lot of blue in nature. The bowers you see today are adorned mainly with blue clothes pegs, plastic straws and the tops off milk bottles.

Once his bower is complete, the male will trill and dance around it in the hope of enticing a willing female. It's hard to see any intrinsic meaning in his collection of blue baubles—they are not in themselves of any use nor is the roofless bower which is built on the ground, with no protection from preda-tors or the elements. The whole exercise only makes sense on a symbolic level. The bower and its ornaments represent the male's power and status within his world, indicating to females how desirable a mate he is. The stronger adult males routinely steal blue trinkets from adolescent birds mak-ing their first ventures into the mating game, thus establishing that they are more powerful. Is it really that different from the man who cruises the streets in an open-top sports car?

Male display for the benefit of choosy females is a feature of the animal world, but it is not the only observation that can be made about non-human sex. In fact, the most striking thing about animals' sexual behavior is how incredibly varied it is between—and sometimes even within—species. Look closely enough and we find pair-bonds that last a lifetime, same-sex encoun-ters, females that mate with males and leave them to raise the babies—a thousand variations that do not always seem to fit terribly well with evolutionary imperatives. A clear model for human sexual behavior is not going to be easy to find.

CHIMP BALLS AND SEAL BLUBBER

"We're *designed* to be promiscuous," says a man I meet at a wedding. "I mean *look* at chimps. Society forces us into these monogamous relationships that are totally at odds with the way we're meant to behave."

Whatever our own pet theory about the essential nature of human beings, of men or women, chances are we'll be able to find an animal model to "prove" it. And the most fertile ground of all for such speculations has to be our closest relatives, the chimpanzees and their cousins, the bonobos. Along with us humans, they, the gorillas, and the orangutans make up the great apes, and we look to these nearest relatives for insights into our own species' behavioral evolution, as anthropologist Craig Stanford explains:

> Chimpanzees and bonobos provide us with examples of the range of possible adaptations for feeding, ranging, territoriality, mating, offspring rearing, and a variety of other behaviors without which there would be no starting point for reconstructing hominid societies.

Chimps live in large groups of perhaps one hundred or more and behaviors vary between groups in different locations, suggesting they, like us, have the capacity to develop different cultures. They are not peaceful creatures, fighting frequently among themselves and engaging in vicious, sometimes lethal, wars with neighboring tribes. Each band has one dominant male, but he is constantly fending off attack from subordinate males and his time at the top is generally brief. Both sexes are highly promiscuous. Although the dominant male will father about half of all young during his brief reign, the females certainly share the love around, mating with various males at a rate that has been estimated at up to one thousand times for every pregnancy. And they don't just stick to their own tribe either. Despite the hostility between males of different bands, the females will sneak off and have furtive sex with the enemy when their own males are not looking.

The lives of bonobos, in contrast, tend to be portrayed as one long, happy orgy. Once known as pygmy chimpanzees, and similar to chimps in appearance, they have only been objects of serious study since the 1980s, and since then they have become known as the "make love, not war" apes. Some observers have described them as engaged in more or less constant sexual activity, heterosexual, homosexual, during their fertile period and outside it, even between adults and young. Female-to-female genital rubbing may be the most common form of sexual activity in the species and appears to be used to cement bonds between females that help them to dominate the males. As primatologist Frans de Waal puts it: "The chimpanzee resolves sexual issues with power; the bonobo resolves power issues with sex." Bonobo females, like chimps, have sex with males from other bands but they are not surreptitious about it, performing the act in full view of their own males. The bonobos don't fight much. They're probably too exhausted. Or perhaps too flooded with pleasure-giving hormones. Here's de Waal again:

> Bonobo society, unlike that of chimpanzees, is best characterized as female centered and egalitarian, with sex substituting for aggression. Females occupy prominent, often ruling positions in society, and the high points of bonobo intellectual life are found not in cooperative hunting or strategies to achieve dominance but in conflict resolution and sensitivity to others.

It's not hard to see why these apes have become pin-up girls for those who seek a gentler model for human societies and relationships between the sexes. We'd probably prefer that our politicians refrained from "resolving power issues with sex," at least in public, but on the whole bonobo society seems like a sort of feminist utopia with loads of action for everybody. Males maintain a close bond with their mothers all their lives and even alpha males have been observed making submissive gestures, such as grinning and bending away, at the approach of a female. Females also control food distribution and often refuse to share an antelope kill or gathered fruit with males. Anthropologist Ellen Ingmanson observed this scene at Wamba in the Congo:

> When a high-ranking adult female . . . captured a flying squirrel, she proceeded to share it with other adult females and their offspring. None of the carcass went to any of the adult males, however, even though the highest-ranking male of the group had a temper tantrum on a branch below the feasting females.

Whether you opt for chimpanzees or bonobos as models for human behavior will probably depend on your own view of the world. If you like the idea of us as a co-operative, sensual, female-dominated species, the bonobos will be likely to appeal. If you prefer to see us as a more aggressive, male-dominated lot, you'll probably go for the chimps.

But, either way, there's always a risk that we're imposing our own desires and preconceptions on the animals when we use them to bolster pet theories of human behavior. Earlier generations of observers tended to look for the nuclear family in nature and, with the focus squarely on male dominance, were often blind to the ways females might exercise power within any animal group. Appealing as the bonobos seem, I can't help wondering if something similar might be happening here, if we are not perhaps looking at these animals through rose-colored glasses in an attempt to find a gentler model for our own interactions with each other.

Stanford indeed suggests anthropologists may have gone too far in idealizing the bonobos, emphasizing their differences from chimps while ignoring the substantial similarities: bonobo males are not always submissive to females and they do fight with each other, albeit not as viciously as chimps, and chimps resemble the bonobos in having sex vigorously and frequently. Some accounts of the two species seem to impose a stereotypical human sex-role binary on the animals, Stanford argues, with the murderous, sexually coercive, status-obsessed chimps representing men while the non-aggressive, sensual, cooperative bonobos represent women: "While these characterizations are based on observational data, they may also be influenced by views of the two apes that accord with human male and female gender stereotypes," he writes.

To demonstrate how subjective our representations of animal behavior can be, Stanford sets out two equally valid ways in which chimpanzee society could be described: as demonstrating male dominance, aggression and coercion toward females who are essentially reproductive commodities for which males compete; or as a mating system driven by promiscuous females who solicit males for sex and incite them to compete with each other around the time of ovulation.

The other two members of the great ape family complicate the picture further. In gorilla bands, the dominant male can remain in control for several years at a time. Because the females are only sexually active occasionally, he does not have to fight to maintain his position all that often. Gorilla bands are generally described as a "harem" controlled by one dominant male, although again this use of a human term to describe animal behavior is problematic. Just as there are several equally valid ways of describing chimpanzee behavior, descriptions of gorilla sexual organization could also be turned on their head and portrayed as the largely self-sufficient females selecting the best equipped male to provide them with sperm when they are ready to mate.

In fact, gorillas provide another reminder of how easy it is for us to overlay our own assumptions onto animal behavior. We see a mighty silverback pounding his chest and we assume the females and subordinate males would never *dare* transgress. But, in fact, DNA tests have recently suggested female gorillas may be more flexible about their partners than previously suspected. Several genetic studies have shown the dominant silverback sires the majority—but not all—offspring in those gorilla groups that include more than one adult male. Researchers from the Max Planck Institute for Evolutionary Anthropology, for example, conducted genetic tests in two mountain gorilla bands living in the wonderfully named Bwindi Impenetrable National Park in southwestern Uganda. It emerged the females were not quite as impenetrable as their home territory, with DNA tests revealing the dominant male sired only five of seven young in one group and eight of ten in the other. How much this genetic diversity results from the patriarch's inability to be watching everybody all of the time, and how much it reflects female preference for another mate is open to interpretation.

Last among our cousins are the orangutans, the red-haired apes that perhaps look most human to us, though are the most distant on the evolutionary tree. Their name in fact means "man of the forest" in Malay. Sadly, the tropical rainforests of Borneo and Sumatra that are their home are retreating before an invading front of palm oil plantations and these great apes, like their African cousins, face serious threats to their survival. Orangutans are the most solitary of the apes, with one male controlling a constantly changing territory, within which live several females each with her own smaller territory, marital arrangements that irresistibly remind me of the HBO television series about a polygamous Mormon family, *Big Love*.

The Sepilok Orang-Utan Rehabilitation Centre in Borneo is one of only four orangutan sanctuaries in the world. Orphaned and injured animals are brought here to be rehabilitated before returning to what is left of the wild. I visit during a tropical monsoon, and low clouds threaten rain as the animals emerge from the rainforest at feeding time, swinging along ropes strung between the trees to the fruit platform. After the meal is over and the shutter-clicking tourists have retreated, I stay on to watch two young orangutans who have not yet headed back into the jungle. The adolescent male is "courting" the female. His approach is to grab hold of her leg as she climbs a tree away from him and try to pull her back down: not a winning strategy. The stand-off lasts for perhaps twenty minutes. With him holding on to her leg, she can't keep climbing, but she's not coming down either. A keeper tells me the female's resistance is because she is still too young to mate. Eventually, the young male gives up and releases her leg. Almost immediately, she comes down the tree of her own accord and the two of them amble off together down the tourist boardwalk. With their stooped posture and shuffling walk, they remind me of an elderly human couple crossing a road. As they walk, he gently places an arm across her back.

And of course I am doing what every observer of the primates seems to do: anthropomorphizing. I find myself imagining that she actually quite likes her suitor but was not coming down from that tree until he backed off and accepted that she would only do this on her terms. And I can't help seeing the gesture with his arm as an expression of . . . *tenderness*. It is hard to look at these animals, so like us in so many ways, and not attribute human motivations and desires to them.

Given how extraordinarily different the social and sexual behaviors of our great ape cousins are, it is no surprise that observers have been able to find support for just about any claims about human behavior by drawing on one or another primary species. As geneticist Steve Jones puts it, even in our closest relatives the "erotic habits are remarkably diverse." And we haven't ventured beyond the great apes to talk about the pair-bonded gibbons or the male-pursuing female langurs. Jones again: "Given the speed at which sex evolves, to search for the remnants of any fundamental rule in such a miscellaneous group may be too much to ask."

In the hunt for evidence about the "nature" of human sexuality, some researchers have therefore resorted to physiology, something that can at least be measured more objectively. Various differences between animals, from body size to the appearance of their genitals, are held to relate to differences in sexual behavior.

This is where the chimp testicles come in. And what testicles they are: if human males had equivalent balls, they'd be the size of grapefruit. Gorillas, in contrast, are under-endowed, with testicles only half the size of humans', relative to body size. What do the testicles mean? The argument is that they are an index of female promiscuity. In species where the girls mate with all and sundry, the boys' main hope of gaining an evolutionary advantage is by producing more copious and more vigorous sperm, hence the larger testicles. So the promiscuous chimp females bring out enormously larger balls in their mates than do the more (though, as we've seen, not entirely) faithful gorillas. Human females, according to this argument, would be as Jones puts it "moderately promiscuous," more so than gorillas, but much less so than chimps.

The other physiological line of thought when it comes to sexual behavior relates to physical differences between males and females within a species (the technical term for this is sexual dimorphism). Usually manifesting as a difference in physical size, sexual dimorphism is considered to be an indicator of polygamy or, more accurately, polygyny, the arrangement that sees one male having more or less exclusive sexual access to several females. Its opposite, polyandry, is rare in the animal world, although it does exist in some species of birds, posing a challenge to the idea that egg producers are hard-wired to focus on quality rather than quantity while sperm producers do the opposite. In some species of shore birds, for example, the larger, more brightly colored females lay a clutch of eggs and leave the father to raise them, while they head off and find a second and even sometimes a third mate.

Polygynous animals tend to show the biggest disparities in size between males and females, the reason being that males in such a system generally use physical battles to demonstrate to the females that they have the best genes. Being bigger and stronger thus gives them an evolutionary advantage that it would not offer their mates. The most extreme example is perhaps the elephant seal, where the extremely aggressive male can weigh up to 3.7 metric tons, as much as four times the size of an adult female. In their vicious fights for supremacy, these huge lumps of blubber thrash about, frequently crushing pups and even adult females to death in the process. One study found that just 4 percent of male elephant seals account for 88 percent of all copulations. In the polygynous gorilla, a large male can be twice the size of a female, whereas in the indiscriminately promiscuous chimpanzees and the pair-bonded gibbons the two sexes are similar in size. Here again, though, there are exceptions to the rule such as horses, which like most grazing animals are polygynous yet show little difference in size between the sexes.

Humans do show some sexual dimorphism, with men on average being taller and stronger than women. However, the difference doesn't come close to that seen in elephant seals and, in fact, the two sexes overlap to a very large extent. Unlike those of the male great apes who fight for access to females, human males also do not have larger canine teeth than females. Evolutionists tend to conclude from the real, but relatively small, differences between men and women that we are a mildly polygynous species, something that seems to be supported by anthropology. Although most human societies seem to have accepted polygamy to some extent, officially or otherwise, it does not ever seem to have been the universal rule—fortunately for men, since a society where all women lived in polygynous relationships would be one in which most men lived lives of quiet desperation. Allowing a small number of males to father the bulk of our infants, as the elephant seals do, would also considerably reduce the creative genetic diversity that is a mark of our species.

It is possible, though, that researchers have not paid enough attention to non-physiological ways in which human sexual dimorphism might be expressed. Heterosexual men and women generally seek similar things in their partners: kindness and fidelity, for example. But there are two main points on which the sexes diverge. Men are more focused on the youth of their partner, with their preferred age gap increasing as they themselves age. And, although it pains me to admit it, studies tend to suggest women find wealthier men more attractive. It is possible that this will change, of course, if female earning power ever equals that of men but, given how long inequalities between the sexes have been with us, it seems at least worth considering that the real human sexual dimorphism is in wealth and power, rather than physical size.

In any case, the distinctions between monogamy and polygamy may not be as clear-cut as we like to imagine. Most humans, at least throughout recorded history, seem to have lived in long-term pair-bonds for purposes of procreation, child rearing, and economic cooperation, but that doesn't mean they never strayed. Again, genetic testing in animals is increasingly revealing that "social monogamy"—the pair-bond—does not necessarily imply sexual monogamy on the part of either females or males. There is mounting evidence that females may choose one male as long-term partner material, while also selecting others purely on genetic merit as sperm donors. Offspring in "monogamous" species as diverse as blackbirds and gibbons have been found to have been sired by a male other than the father who has raised them. Of course, these "wives" could only be playing away if the "husbands" of other females were also up for it, so it's not a question of making one sex out to be more dissolute than the other.

So has the wedding guest proved his point and were we designed for promiscuity? The range of behaviors and systems of sexual organization found in animals and our own societies seems to rule out a simple answer to such a question. In fact, I find myself wondering about this whole idea of looking for humans' "natural" sexual behavior. Why do we assume that the way we behave now is *not* natural? We seem to see ourselves as a sort of bipedal version of chimpanzees in captivity, our behaviors perverted by an artificial environment. Unlike the chimps, though, our cage—society—is one we have designed and built ourselves, making it arguably as good a representation of our natures as anything else.

Perhaps the main reason we turn to the animals for answers is that we are hoping to find a simpler picture than we can ever get from looking at ourselves. If animal sexual behavior is complex and confusing, ours is a great deal more so. From shoe fetishism to erotic auto-asphyxiation, humans display a huge array of behaviors, many of which do not sit easily with theories of evolutionary advantage. But it seems to me that maybe this *is* our nature: to indulge in a wide variety of sexual practices for a multitude of reasons, only some of which relate to procreation. Like the chimps, we can be promiscuous and can fight with each other over opportunities to mate. Like the gibbons, we sometimes mate for life. Like the gorillas, our most powerful males sometimes enjoy access to multiple partners (though they may also be deceived about those partners' fidelity). And like the bonobos, we see sex as not just procreative, but also as a way of creating bonds between individuals, whether of the same sex or different ones.

DOMESTICATING HUMANS

One of the key claims of evolutionary psychology is that we are all essentially unchanged since the Pleistocene but, in fact, there is evidence that under the right circumstances evolution can move surprisingly quickly.

In 1959, Russian geneticist Dimitry Belyaev set out to understand how a species might evolve in the process of becoming domesticated. At Novosibirsk in Siberia, he began breeding captive silver foxes for a single behavioral trait: tameness. By mating the tamest male and female in each generation with each other, he produced *within twenty years* animals that were dramatically different both physically and behaviorally from those he began with. He produced, in fact, foxes that behaved like domestic dogs, actively seeking human company and wagging their tails when approached. Their coat color changed, their ears became floppy rather than pricked, new vocal calls appeared, hormone levels changed and they started breeding outside the normal mating season. Intriguingly, there was some evidence of a reduction in physical differences between the sexes, as the shape of the males' skulls became more like that of the females. Belyaev's colleague Lyudmila Trut wrote after his death:

> By intense selective breeding, we have compressed into a few decades what originally unfolded over thousands of years. Before our eyes . . . the aggressive behavior of our herd's wild progenitors entirely disappeared.

Evolutionary biologist Richard Dawkins has pointed out that we generally have different words for the wild and tame versions of species that have most closely shared our lives over recent millennia: wolves and dogs, for example. It is obvious that we humans have had a major impact on the genes of many plants and other animals, in some cases through selective breeding as in the silver fox experiment, in others through these species finding an evolutionary advantage in interactions with us. The myriad of dog breeds we see today may be largely a result of deliberate breeding by humans, but the first evolutionary step in domesticating the wolf was probably taken when those wild animals that were less scared of humans prospered because proximity to our camps gave them easier access to food.

It is less common for us to consider the impact close contact with other species might have had on our own genes. We do not, as Dawkins puts it, have a word for the domesticated version of the human species, but it "seems plausible that we ourselves evolved down a parallel road of domestication after the Agricultural Revolution, towards our own version of tameness and associated by-product traits." Researchers have recently, in fact, found evidence of evolutionary changes in our species over the last ten thousand years or so in areas as diverse as diet, skin pigment, sense of smell, fertility, and brain development. This is still very much a work in progress (as are we, in evolutionary terms), with researchers still trying to pin down exactly what may have changed and why.

Perhaps one of the most striking examples of our domestication can be found in lactose tolerance, an adaptation not found in all modern humans but seemingly concentrated in those with a history of pastoralism. Mammals generally are not designed to digest dairy products beyond the age when they are weaned, at which point the gene that produces the milk-digesting enzyme lactase is normally switched off. In humans, this happens at about age four.

However, some of us have evolved so that the gene does not get switched off, a genetic change that has been driven by a change in culture, as Dawkins explains:

> The evolution of tameness and increasing milk yields in cattle, sheep and goats paralleled that of lactose tolerance in the tribes that herded them. Both were true evolutionary trends in that they were changes in gene frequencies in populations. But both were driven by non-genetic cultural changes.

If we can evolve to be able to digest milk products into adulthood, what other genetic changes might not have happened in response to cultural changes, he goes on to ask:

> Is lactose tolerance just the tip of the iceberg? Are our genomes riddled with evidences of domestication, affecting not just our biochemistry but our minds? . . . [L]ike the domesticated wolves that we call dogs, have we become tamer, more lovable, with the human equivalents of floppy ears, soppy faces and wagging tails?

Does this mean our genes could have evolved along with our cultures more generally, albeit with a considerable time lag? Our complex societies—whether based on a hunter-gatherer or agricultural economic model—would certainly have imposed different evolutionary imperatives on us from those experienced by the first "wild" humans. We might speculate, for example, that greater ability to control an aggressive response would become an evolutionary advantage as social controls increased, where the opposite might have been true in the earliest human societies. And, given that the pair-bond has been a feature of so many societies, perhaps we have also evolved to fit its imperatives, with both sexes selecting mates for qualities such as loyalty and fidelity as well as reproductive health or physical strength. If children from stable relationships are more likely to survive to reproductive age, then this would further reinforce the passing on of such genes.

Nobody has yet identified a "fidelity gene," and it's doubtful such complex behaviors could be entirely explained by a single gene, or even by many genes acting together. We might have a genetic predisposition to being faithful, perhaps, but our actual behavior would depend on a huge number of unpredictable interactions between our genes and other aspects of our biology and environment.

We do know, though, that the pace of evolution can speed up dramatically when a particular quality—physical or behavioral—comes to be seen as desirable in a potential mate. So, if humans at some point in our history had begun to see sexual fidelity as an important quality, it is conceivable that we could have evolved quite quickly to become more faithful. The reason this process of "sexual selection" can promote faster evolution is that individuals who lack the valued quality may have difficulty finding a mate at all, while those who are well endowed may be extremely successful. If everybody in the world decided tomorrow that red-headed people were not suitable sexual partners, for example, the trait would almost disappear from the world within a generation. Equally, if the whole world decided some random quality like the ability to wiggle your earlobes was irresistibly attractive, we could expect this skill to become far more prevalent within very few generations.

Of course, fashions in attractiveness are never as universal as this, fortunately for most of us, but sexual selection does offer a potential mechanism for incorporating cultural change into the evolutionary process. It is possible to speculate that women in more lawless times might have placed a higher value on physical strength in a mate as a representation of his ability to protect them from danger. As that quality has become less useful in our more managed societies, have we perhaps begun to select against it and in favor of other traits that are more useful in a modern man?

Sexual selection can sometimes seem bizarre in its effects, creating what Dawkins describes as "rapid, apparently arbitrary spurts of evolution in quirky directions." While many of the qualities one sex finds attractive in the other are good indicators of general or reproductive health, some really do seem to be just random expressions of fashion. Perhaps the best example of this is the peacock's tail. Peahens choose their mates based on the size and splendor of this appendage, and the males of the species have therefore evolved to grow ever larger and more cumbersome adornments. Scientists have devoted considerable time to attempts to understand why such an impediment to easy movement, and therefore to survival, should have been favored by evolution, with suggestions ranging from the idea that any male who survived *in spite* of his burden would be considered exceptionally strong to its being simply a question of female taste.

Whatever its origins, when a trait like the peacock's tail becomes sexually attractive, there is an inbuilt tendency for that preference to be perpetuated. The peahen who chooses the partner with the biggest tail will pass on to her offspring of both sexes not only their father's big tail genes but also any genes that encode her own preference for big tails. So the next generation will be more likely to have big tails if male and more likely to prefer them in partners if female, leading to what Dawkins calls "runaway evolution."

In fact, Dawkins has wondered if sexual selection might lie behind our own evolutionary divergence from the other apes, as we became bipedal, hairless, and brainy. Could it be that humans of both sexes selected mates for intelligence, leading to a rapid expansion in brain size and functioning? Speed of movement and sheer brute strength would have been important qualities in our hunter-gatherer ancestors, but it is likely they also valued mates who were smart, those who were particularly good, for example, at working out and remembering where particular animal or vegetable foods could be found and under what weather conditions. Our brains could be the human equivalent of the peacock's tail. Rather than splaying our feathers to attract a mate, we talk, tell jokes, invent useful contraptions or create works of art.

Biologist Anne Fausto-Sterling has suggested one of the defining qualities of the human genome may be that it is designed for flexibility and adaptability rather than to force us down predetermined behavioral paths, and here too our brains would be key. If she is right, this might help to explain the bewildering diversity of human cultures despite our all sharing very similar genes.

In her work as an animal biologist, Fausto-Sterling has observed that species that evolve to fit their environment too neatly can actually be doing themselves a disservice. "The more perfectly adapted an organism is to its environment, the less flexibility it has should the environment change," she writes, citing the "shy and environmentally limited" Californian condor as an example of an animal under threat.

Other species, however, evolve to be pests. Think invasive weeds, raccoons, possums, and . . . perhaps humans. Precisely because these species have adapted less successfully to a particular ecological niche, they are able to prosper in a variety of environments. So both the American raccoon and the Australian possum have become successful urban scavengers following the widespread disappearance of their forest habitat.

Maybe it's not too big a stretch to suggest that the very fact that our species has managed to populate the globe from the frozen Arctic to tropical islands, and has produced so many different and such rapidly changing cultures along the way, suggests our distant ancestors did not in fact adapt narrowly to their original home on the savannah. Rather than men evolving to be hunters and women to be communal child nurturers, it seems more likely that both sexes evolved to be flexible, creative, and quick to respond to unfamiliar challenges. Perhaps it is our ability to adopt new behaviors in response to changing circumstances that is truly hard-wired into our psyches, helping to explain the huge shift in sex roles we have seen over the last half-century and perhaps even our success as a species.

Chapter Three

Hermes and Aphrodite

Argentinian writer Jorge Luis Borges wrote in one of his essays about "a certain Chinese encyclopaedia" in which animals were classified into the following categories:

> (a) those that belong to the Emperor, (b) embalmed ones, (c) those that are trained, (d) suckling pigs, (e) mermaids, (f) fabulous ones, (g) stray dogs, (h) those that are included in this classification, (i) those that tremble as if they were mad, (j) innumerable ones, (k) those drawn with a very fine camel's hair brush, (l) others, (m) those that have just broken a flower vase, (n) those that resemble flies from a distance.

French philosopher Michel Foucault said he laughed out loud when he first read this passage and so did I. There is something irresistibly funny about such unrelated categories as "suckling pigs" and "those that have broken a flower vase" being placed in a list as though they represent equivalent, and equally valuable, ways of understanding the nature of things. It is a magnificent, subversive parody of the scientific project of ordering and classifying the world. So perhaps it is no surprise that somebody whose very existence challenges our desire for neat categories should include a link to Foucault's comments on her website.

I meet Bonnie Hart on a cool day at the end of a Sydney summer. The thirty-something artist is passing through town in an unreliable car full of musical equipment and agrees to spend an hour at a café before starting the long drive back to her hometown of Melbourne. She is already at a table when I arrive: an attractive, auburn-haired woman in a red jacket and sunglasses she describes as her "La Dolce Vita look."

I'm in the final stages of writing this book and I've interviewed scientists and clinicians who work with ambiguities of biological sex, but this is the first time an intersex person has been willing to meet me to talk about their experiences. I've sent emails to various groups around the world and my contact details have been posted in newsletters and discussion groups, but the most I've had up till now has been the occasional message of encouragement accompanied by a polite refusal.

Hart is understandably cautious. She spends some time questioning me about my motives, having previously made it clear she will not participate in any "damaging eugenics bio-nightmare." As somebody who embraces the word "hermaphrodite," finding it more poetic and other-worldly than the more commonly used "intersex," she is keen to combat the culture of secrecy and shame that can surround people in her position. Although others in her Catholic extended family shared her genetic condition, it was rarely talked about and Hart herself did not reveal her status to anybody outside the family until she was nineteen: "I developed a really intense lying methodology," she says. "Like, I was *coerced* into that in order to not disclose. I had to lie a lot about things in order to not let the truth out."

Hart and her older sister both have androgen insensitivity syndrome (AIS). Their XY chromosomes meant they developed testes that produced normal male levels of testosterone but a glitch in the androgen receptors meant their bodies were unable to "read" the hormone. This inability to use male hormones means people with AIS switch to a female developmental path in utero. Their external appearance and gender identity is generally female but, in the absence of ovaries and a uterus, these women cannot have children. They also have little or no pubic and underarm hair because this requires the participation of testosterone in both sexes. AIS is often not identified until puberty when a girl is taken to a doctor to see why her period has not arrived, although in Hart's case the family history meant her testes were noticed soon after birth.

Like many girls with AIS, she had those testes surgically removed in childhood, something she is still angry about. "They were *my* testes," she says emphatically. "If they weren't broken, then why get rid of them?" Although undescended testes do carry an increased cancer risk, Hart believes this could have been addressed by careful monitoring and the gonads might have provided her with a natural source of other hormones such as estrogen that could have reduced her reliance on supplements.

She suspects one reason some doctors may be, as she puts it, "knife happy" is their own discomfort at the presence of a male organ such as a testis in an otherwise female body (or, for example, a clitoris the size of a penis on a baby classified as female). Rather than using surgery to "normalize" children with ambiguous genitals, she would like to see society accept that people like her have a unique perspective on the world that should be valued as it is. In tribal societies, people who existed outside the conventional sex binary ("if they weren't infanticided" for being different) might have occupied special positions as shamans or healers, she says. "Why say it's wrong and give it words like abnormality? It's just so perverse really, worrying about this thing rather than embracing it." Yes, people can be cruel to those who are perceived as different, but, "Why should such brutality, the fear of somebody acting like a bigoted moron, deem what is acceptable or the social norm?"

Like many intersex people, Hart has also struggled with the effects of being an object of scientific curiosity from early childhood on. "Everyone wants to rubberneck at the AIS person," she says. Although she understands medical students have to be trained, she wonders if this couldn't have been better handled. "I have memories of being a young child with my legs spread on a metal table with about 15 student doctors standing around. And one doctor saying, 'Now, if I put my finger in here.'" She laughs as she imitates the jocular male voice of the finger's owner and at the memory of her childhood self involuntarily releasing a fart at its approach.

Because girls with AIS generally have short, blind-ending vaginas, they also can face surgery designed to facilitate penetrative sex. The option was discussed during Hart's childhood but, to her relief, never proceeded with, although she was made to perform unpleasant and she believes unnecessary vaginal stretching exercises. "I was like in sexual training from when I was 12 or 11, which was pretty radically *young*," Hart says. "I was told by doctors that I would never be able to have normal penetrative sex unless I used like these *dilators* and stuff like that. It was like one day *maybe* I'll be able to accommodate the future partner that doesn't even exist yet and in the meantime I'll make out with this thing that looks like a mop handle!? Do you know what I mean!? It was totally detached from sensuality, like the idea of sexuality being just automated pump and grind."

Although she identifies as and looks female, Hart says she tends not to use the word "woman" to describe herself. "A woman is more than an adult female," she says. "At least in the cultural terminology. Like, I don't have a female internal reproductive system. I don't menstruate. . . . Someone asked me why I would deny myself that title and I'm like, well, do I need a label?"

I suggest it's perhaps a question of how she feels and she stares at me blankly.

"I don't *know* what I feel. I mean, like, what's normal? It's easier to label something and that way it's labeled, pre-defined, but then that doesn't allow the thing to change. It doesn't allow it to morph or grow." In a similar vein, she's been asked whether she thinks like a man or a woman but, as she says, how would she know? "I just think how I think."

And that way of thinking is definitely individual. As she sips her tea, Hart's conversation leaps from one idea to the next with exhilarating, often bewildering, speed. Topics covered include black holes, quantum physics, and whether gravity might one day decide to stop being constant; her expectation that multitudes of emancipated hermaphrodites will one day challenge the status quo; how horrible it must be for computer programmers to be immersed all day in a binary world; the limitations of the theory of evolution and her desire for a model that is based on cooperation rather than competition; and the possible existence of a three-meter-long "flailing clitoris." At one point, she draws breath and apologizes for the deluge: "Sorry, flooding . . ."

Her lively unpredictable take on the world is, Hart believes, in part a product of her unusual biological status: "If you are conventionally, historically, said not to exist and then, when you do exist, you exist as a freak that needs to be normalized, then you *have* to ask questions about the system of thought that says you don't exist," she says. "And it's full of holes."

BEYOND THE BINARY

If anything highlights the impossibility of finding a cast-iron definition of the two sexes, it is those people whose anatomy does not neatly fit into one category or the other. People with ambiguous external genitalia used to be put on display in traveling shows, along with bearded ladies, captured pygmies, Siamese twins, and other so-called freaks of nature. We tend to think we've come a long way since then, though observers of the furor that engulfed Caster Semenya could have had their doubts.

AIS is only one of a mixed bunch of intersex conditions that affect a surprisingly large number of people. Just how many is difficult to say: incidence varies in different populations and there is no universal agreement on what should be included in the definition. As a result, estimates vary hugely, from one in 4,500 newborns in the Western world to as many as one in fifty. Geneticist Eric Vilain from the University of California in Los Angeles has estimated that about one in one hundred babies born in Western countries has atypical genitals at birth, although not all of these children would necessarily be classified as intersex. The figure includes those with enlarged clitorises, small penises, a misplaced urethral opening or undescended testes. But even the lower estimate of one in 4500 makes intersex conditions more common than better known "birth defects," such as Down's syndrome.

I'm struggling with language here. Many intersex people are angered by descriptions of their anatomy as a defect or disorder, seeing it rather as a normal variation. They campaign vocally to be accepted as they are and against surgery being performed on children before they are able to consent unless this is essential for medical reasons. The word "intersex" is itself a contested one—clinicians often prefer to talk about disorders of sexual development (DSDs)—but I have chosen to use the term, believing it to be the one least likely to offend those it describes.

Some researchers believe intersex conditions are on the rise due to the wash of chemicals that surrounds us. Geneticist Peter Koopman warns over lunch in his institute's café that the presence of so many endocrine (hormonal system) disruptors in the modern world could pose a serious threat to the fertility of our species:

> There's a huge crisis looming . . . these disrupting chemicals can be in *anything*—we're not sure *what* they are so we're not sure *where* they are. They seem to be small chemical molecules that either mimic hormones, or block hormone receptors, or have some other influence on hormone pathways. It's not just the oestrogens in your soy latte. They could be in your shoe polish. They could be in your floor cleaner. Anything that you bring into the home with your shopping, or are exposed to at work, that isn't purely 100 percent natural. Insecticides, fertilizers, plastics, deodorants, air fresheners, cleansers of any type, disinfectants. Any food that you eat that hasn't come straight out of the ground or out of a tree. Do you ever eat corn chips? You know those ones that are nachos-flavored and they're *bright red*. There's a sub-stratum of corn and then there's this fluorescent coating of chemical shit. Have you got any idea what's in your lipstick? Whatever it is, it's sitting there on your lips all day and going straight into your digestive system. You buy a car, it smells of plastic for the first six months, all those fumes going into your and your kids' lungs. You work in a building that's air-conditioned—you have no control over what's coming through the air con. The potential exposure to chemicals of unknown effect on endocrine function is absolutely boundless. It is truly frightening because a lot of these endocrine pathways involved in sex development are extremely sensitive and very easily upset.

Scientists have suggested hormonal disruptors and pesticides could be behind the significant increase over recent decades in hypospadias, one of the most common birth defects in boys. Boys with the condition have a sometimes small or curved penis with the urethral opening on the underside rather than at the tip. Hypospadias is often considered an intersex condition, at least in its more severe form when the unfused urethral folds leave the underside of the penis resembling the labia minora of a baby girl's vulva (the name is a compound of two Greek words meaning "beneath" and "tear"). Baby boys with the condition generally have surgery to reposition the urethral opening at the tip of the penis.

Whether other intersex conditions are on the increase is harder to say because records are not kept consistently around the world and some conditions are extremely rare. In fact, it has been suggested that it is wrong to lump all the intersex conditions together as they often have little in common in terms of causes and outcomes. Some intersex people are identified at birth because their external genitals cannot be clearly defined as belonging to one sex or the other. Others may appear externally to be a typical member of one sex but have internal sexual organs of the other or chromosomes that are inconsistent with their biological sex. In some cases, a person's intersex status may not be recognized until they reach adulthood and are unable to conceive or impregnate their partner. On top of that, different cultures vary in what they accept as "normal." Just how big does a girl's clitoris need to be before it will be seen as a problem? Or how small a boy's penis?

Causes of the conditions vary too. They may be genetic, hormonal or some kind of combination of the two. Genetic variations can arise during the division of the primordial germ cell to create two sperm or eggs, a process described in chapter 1: when the two new germ cells swap genetic material, it is possible for genes, or even whole chromosomes, to end up in an unexpected place. One germ cell can end up with one or more extra sex chromosomes while another can be left without any. If such germ cells end up forming an embryo, it can result in a boy who is, for example, XXY or XYY or a girl with only a single X chromosome.

About one in a thousand males is estimated to have one or more extra X chromosomes in a condition known as Klinefelter's syndrome. This condition is not always included in intersex classifications, although those affected generally have small testes that are unlikely to produce sperm and secrete only low levels of testosterone. They may also have a smaller than average penis, scarce body hair and some breast development. Slight intellectual disability is common and increases with each additional X chromosome a man has.

At the other end of the spectrum are women with Turner's syndrome who inherit only one X chromosome, most commonly from their mother. This has been described as "the most common chromosomal abnormality in humans," affecting one in a hundred at conception. However, since almost all affected embryos will spontaneously miscarry, the incidence at birth is only one in ten thousand. Women with Turner's syndrome are usually severely intellectually disabled and are rarely fertile because their eggs, and ovaries, rapidly degenerate, generally before they reach puberty.

Errors during creation of the germ cells can also result in the male *SRY* gene ending up on the wrong chromosome, leading to a boy being born with two X chromosomes or a girl with one X and one Y, as we saw in chapter 1. One doctor tells me about a patient who came to see him because "the guys at the gym" had told him he was a bit weedy looking and suggested he see somebody about getting testosterone. Genetic testing revealed this man had unsuspected female XX chromosomes and, as his gym companions had guessed, very low levels of testosterone. Because the *SRY* gene had found its way onto his paternal X chromosome, he had developed as a male in utero and had gone through a normal male puberty.

Other genetic variations exist too, including a man who inherited an X chromosome from his mother that included the *SRY* gene. He had no idea he was carrying a double dose of the male gene until he passed the chromosome on, fathering two XX children with male traits.

Perhaps even rarer are those people—known in scientific circles as chimaeras, from the figure in Greek mythology with a lion's head, goat's body and serpent's tail—who are created by the merging together of genetic material from more than one fertilized egg. This may happen when two early embryos fuse together to form one individual, although sometimes twins will also swap genetic material through the placenta. Where two embryos of different sexes cleave together, this can result in an individual who is XX in some cells and XY in others. Surprisingly, although such babies can be intersex, most of these embryos develop as unambiguously male, perhaps because the Sertoli cell hit squads we met in chapter 1 effectively wipe out any cells that attempt to get ovarian development going.

Apart from chromosomal variations, the other main cause of intersex conditions is hormonal. This can relate to over- or underexposure to sex hormones or, as in the case of AIS, to the body's ability or inability to make effective use of circulating hormones. While people with complete androgen insensitivity develop a clearly female appearance, those with partial insensitivity can end up looking quite ambiguous.

One of the more common hormone-related conditions is congenital adrenal hyperplasia, in which a baby girl is "masculinized" by high levels of male hormones in utero. Most often this is because her own adrenal gland has been hyperactive in producing androgens, but similar cases have also been observed in baby girls whose mothers were exposed to masculinizing hormones during pregnancy. Girls with the condition may be born with an enlarged, penis-like clitoris, labia majora that have fused together like a scrotal sac and an incompletely formed vagina. They will, however, have ovaries and internal female organs and are usually treated with hormones to support a female sex assignment. Medical opinion on the advisability of early genital surgery in such cases varies, although pediatric endocrinologist Garry Warne tells me he supports it because vaginal reconstruction is more successful when undertaken before too much growth has occurred and the evidence shows these children will identify as female provided hormonal treatment is maintained.

One of the more dramatic intersex conditions is described in Jeffrey Eugenides's novel, *Middlesex*, which tells the story of a little girl called Callie who more or less turns into a boy at puberty. This is not just a novelist's fancy. Callie has a rare intersex condition that, like AIS, sees an XY baby unable to use androgens in the usual way. However, in this case, the mechanism is different and as a result so are the effects. The embryo lacks an enzyme called 5-alpha reductase, which is responsible for turning testosterone into its derivative, dihydrotestosterone, the substance that actually does most of the work of directing male fetal development. So, although the baby has internal testes and normal testosterone levels, the external genitals often look female at birth, albeit possibly with an enlarged clitoris. Around the time of puberty, though, something remarkable happens. The masculinizing changes that happen at that point do not depend on dihydrotestosterone, but directly on testosterone itself, so the child, who may have been considered a girl up to that point, will go through a male puberty. His voice will drop, he will start to grow facial hair and male musculature, his testes may descend into what were thought to be the labia majora and his phallus will enlarge further, though it will probably never achieve the dimensions of a typical penis.

This rare condition clusters in a small number of populations around the world, particularly where close relatives have interbred. (Callie in *Middlesex* is the product of grandparents who are siblings and parents who are first cousins.) In the Dominican Republic, where one such cluster exists, affected children are known as *guevedoche* or "balls at twelve." In the isolated highlands of Papua New Guinea, the Sambia people call boys who they identify with the condition at birth *kwolu-aatmwol* or "changing from a female thing into a male thing." As anthropologist Gilbert Herdt documented, all Sambia boys perform fellatio on adult males as part of puberty rituals, but the kwolu-aatmwol boys do this for longer in the belief it will help to bring out their inner maleness. Although the Sambia have found a place for these children in their culture, it does not seem to be one of total acceptance: the boys are not allowed to participate in the full range of adult male rituals and those who were assigned a female sex at birth occupy an uneasy space, being forbidden male puberty rituals and denied male status in spite of their appearance.

RESTORING ORDER

Western culture has generally been much less accepting of sexual ambiguity than the Sambia appear to be. Our desire for clear categories has seen science search for an unambiguous definition of each individual's one "true sex" even in cases where this seemed an impossible goal. In the past, at least, this seems to have resulted partly from a moral panic about homosexuality: if you can't be sure whether somebody is a man or a woman, how can you determine who it is acceptable for them to have sexual relations with?

Historian Alice Domurat Dreger has documented the struggle of late nineteenth-century European science to come to grips with the troubling figure of the "hermaphrodite." The voyeuristic fascination men of science showed for cases of what was often called "doubtful sex" can be seen in medical texts. The *British Medical Journal*, for example, reported in 1882 on a meeting that discussed one baby:

> Mr. Brian Rigden showed a [subject of] Spurious Hermaphroditism, seven months old. There was a large clitoris, not perforated, and labia without testicles. A small opening existed beneath the clitoris. . . . There was no visible vagina, and the finger in the rectum failed to detect an uterus. . . . This child was considered a female by the meeting. A very amusing and interesting discussion followed.

Science of the time tended to see the female of the species as a less evolved creature than the male, leading to a tendency to view hermaphrodites as either underdeveloped males or overdeveloped females. Although some scientists attempted biological explanations for such irregularities, many also blamed the psychological state of the pregnant woman. Parisian surgeon Jean Samuel Pozzi, for example, did not doubt that "the influence of strong emotions on the production of monstrosities seems established by very strong proofs." Women were indeed warned against looking at any kind of monster while pregnant for fear such unpleasant sights would become imprinted on their unborn child. The 1908 instructional manual, *What a Young Wife Ought to Know* by Emma Drake (MD), commented on the striking resemblance of Italian babies to pictures of baby Jesus caused by the hours their mothers had spent contemplating images of the Madonna and went on to warn:

> Look at beautiful pictures, study perfect pieces of statuary, forbid as far as possible the contemplation of unsightly and imperfect models.

No prizes for guessing that it would be unwise for a pregnant woman to visit a freak show.

With no knowledge of genes and little understanding of the endocrine system, science struggled to find ways of classifying people with confusing anatomy. Dreger has dubbed the late nineteenth century "the age of gonads" because of the increasing reliance on these organs as indicators of an individual's "true" sex. No matter how female (or male) somebody looked or felt, the most reliable definition of their sex was to be based on whether they had testes or ovaries. The advantage of this method was that it provided a clear answer for almost everybody. People may have all kinds of ambiguities in their physical appearance but so-called "true hermaphroditism"—still today defined as the presence of both ovarian and testicular tissue in the one body—is rare. All others, like the baby who made that brief appearance in the *British Medical Journal*, were defined as pseudohermaphrodites. The troubling figure of the hermaphrodite was being eliminated, not by eugenics, but by defining such people out of existence.

Given that doctors back then lacked noninvasive technologies for looking inside people's bodies, there was still a fair bit of guesswork involved. A lot of medical fingers were poked up rectums to palpate unseen internal structures in the hope of declaring the presence or absence of a testis, ovary, or uterus. Medical men, in fact, engaged in debates over whether a simple digital examination sufficed or whether the insertion of the whole hand was required.

Vestiges of the classifying work done by these early medical men remain with us today, particularly in the term pseudohermaphroditism, which still crops up in the scientific literature despite being considered offensive by many intersex people. ("You can't even be a real hermaphrodite, man! Shit, can't get *anything* right," says Bonnie Hart.) True hermaphroditism is rare, scientists will tell you, because it requires the presence of either an ovary on one side and a testis on the other or an ovotestis, a single organ that contains both ovarian and testicular tissue.

As the twentieth century advanced, the medical approach to sexual ambiguity became more ambitious. Better understanding of the endocrine system—of hormones—and improved surgical techniques began to open up the possibility of bringing recalcitrant bodies into line. It's not hard to understand why clinicians, and indeed parents, might have thought giving their child a body that belonged clearly to one sex or the other would give them the best chance of happiness. In a world that gives such a central place to gender as a component of identity, the thought of raising a child who is not clearly one thing or the other arouses fears that they might be bullied at school, discriminated against at work, and find themselves unable to form a relationship. With the wisdom of hindsight, though, some of the interventions undertaken a generation or so ago in the belief they would give children a better chance of a "normal" life seem horrifying.

Particularly striking was the centrality of the penis to clinical decision-making. It was pretty much standard practice until at least the 1970s to turn intersex babies whose penises were deemed inadequate into girls, removing or downsizing the organ and providing female hormones in the apparent belief that nobody could be a man without a fully fledged phallus. From a surgical point of view, it is easier to construct a vagina than a penis—or, as Hart graphically puts it, "They used to say it was easier to dig a hole than to make a pole." As recently as 1993, a paper in the *European Journal of Pediatrics* said, "The decision to raise the child as a male centers around the potential for the phallus to function adequately in later sexual relations." And a 1992 urology textbook echoed Hart, albeit in more proper language: "Because it is simpler to construct a vagina than a satisfactory penis, only the infant with a phallus of adequate size should be considered for a male gender assignment."

One of the justifications for turning boys into girls was the belief that infants were a blank slate when it came to gender identity. Key to this argument was the famous John/Joan case, which we'll come back to in more detail in chapter 5. In the mid-1960s, a baby boy code-named "John" had his penis accidentally burned off during a procedure to relieve an over-tight foreskin. Clinicians in Baltimore advised he be reassigned as a female with the assistance of surgery and hormonal treatment. So John became Joan. For this particular child, the results were ultimately shown to have been catastrophic, but for years the so-called successful reassignment was trumpeted as "proof" such interventions worked.

In recent decades, many intersex people have borne witness to the catastrophic effects such medical treatments have had on their lives. Here is Cheryl Chase, the founder of the Intersex Society of North America and the world's best known intersex advocate, writing about her "career as a hermaphrodite":

> I was born [in the 1950s] with ambiguous genitals. A doctor specializing in intersexuality deliberated for three days—sedating my mother each time she asked what was wrong with her baby—before concluding that I was male, with a micropenis, complete hypospadias, undescended testes, and a strange extra opening behind the urethra. A male birth certificate was completed for me, and my parents began raising me as a boy. When I was a year and a half old my parents consulted a different set of experts, who admitted me to a hospital for "sex determination." . . . They judged my genital appendage to be inadequate as a penis, too short to mark masculine status effectively or to penetrate females. As a female, however, I would be penetrable and potentially fertile. My anatomy having been relabeled as vagina, urethra, labia, and outsized clitoris, my sex was determined . . . by amputating my genital appendage. Following doctors' orders, my parents then changed my name, combed their house to eliminate all traces of my existence as a boy (photographs, birthday cards, etc.), changed my birth certificate, moved to a different town, instructed extended family members no longer to refer to me as a boy, and never told anyone else—including me—just what had happened.

As Chase's account shows, even the name given to a child's genitals can vary depending on observers' beliefs about the child's sex. The same organ was described in her case as both a penis and a clitoris, with the choice of label depending entirely on the sex assigned to its owner at that time. Ultimately, the ambiguity was removed along with the organ itself.

Chase's surgical experiences did not end there. At age eight, she returned to the hospital to have the testicular portion of her ovotestes removed, although nobody told her that was what was happening. In adolescence, she began to menstruate but became aware she had no clitoris or labia minora and was unable to have an orgasm. When, after a three-year battle, she obtained her medical records in adulthood, Chase initially saw herself as a monster and contemplated suicide, but eventually found a way out through political activism and the building of an intersex community. She and others began campaigning against pediatric surgery (except when required for medical reasons such as blocked or painful urination), while advocating that children should be raised as either boys or girls, "according to which designation seems likely to offer the child the greatest future sense of comfort."

Although intersex advocates continue to protest against some aspects of medical treatment, there is evidence health professionals have listened. Current guidelines advocate a cautious approach to surgery in childhood and gender assignment is based on a much broader range of factors than the simple presence or absence of an "adequate" penis. Full disclosure of clinical details is advocated for families and, once they are old enough to understand, intersex children.

"There has been a lot of change since I started in medicine," says Warne, who has been practicing in this field for more than thirty years and says he knows of no more vexed area in medical practice. "Our aim really is to have a person whose gender identity matches their genitalia and who is as healthy as they can possibly be. But I think it's important to say that there is no perfect outcome and a lot of the advocates have got themselves wound up because they believe the Holy Grail is the perfect outcome that they never had and were denied by these rotten doctors. They don't understand that things have actually changed a lot. They'd probably be reasonably happy with a lot that we do if they knew about it.

"I think what we're working towards is being able to give an accurate diagnosis more often and taking an approach that is more conservative with regard to surgical intervention, thinking more about what fertility might be enhanced, thinking more about what sexual or other counseling we might have to provide, thinking more about long-term follow-up and support."

He pauses.

"And thinking about how to help the wounded adults out there who have not had the advantage of all that."

Chapter Four

The Sexed Brain

All those psychologists who have studied the intelligence of women, apart from the novelists and poets, recognize today that they represent the most inferior forms of human evolution and are much closer to children and savages than to the civilized adult man. They share with the former changeability, inconstancy, the absence of reflection and logic, the inability to reason or to be influenced by reason, improvidence and the habit of being guided only by the instinct of the moment. . . . One cannot deny, of course, that there exist highly distinguished women, who are greatly superior to the average man, but these are cases as exceptional as the birth of a monstrosity of any kind, such as, for example, a gorilla with two heads, and are in consequence of no relevance whatsoever.

When Parisian craniologist Gustave LeBon wrote these words in the *Revue d'Anthropologie* in 1879, his conclusions were pretty representative of mainstream science. The inferior intelligence of women—along with that of other groups such as "savages" and, often, the working classes—was taken as self-evident. The task of science was simply to reveal the extent of the differences between civilized white men and all the other deficient human beings on the planet. As LeBon put it, "This inferiority [of women's intelligence] is too obvious to be contested even for a moment and one can only debate its degree."

In his quest to provide a scientific basis for woman's intellectual short-comings, LeBon believed the answer would be found in the size of the brain. His mentor, Dr. Paul Broca, had weighed hundreds of them to obtain proof that men's superior intelligence was a result of their larger brains. In the way of early men of science, Broca had an impressively broad intellectual range, managing to be a practicing neurologist, professor in the Paris medical school, director of the school of anthropology, editor of the anthropology journal that published LeBon's research and, before he was carried off by a brain aneurysm, a French senator.

His name is well known to students of brain anatomy for his discovery of the "language center" still known as Broca's area. The first of the many brains he dissected in the service of this discovery, that of a Monsieur Leborgne who was paralyzed down the right side of his body and had lost the power of speech, still swims in a glass jar in what has to be one of the world's strangest museums. Housed in a few hidden-away rooms of the Paris medical school, the nineteenth-century Musée Dupuytren, also known as the museum of pathological anatomy, is home to preserved conjoined twins, wax models of hermaphroditic genitals, and a hallucinatory display of tumors in jars.

LeBon built on Broca's research into female intelligence, or rather the lack of it, by also examining the skulls of inferior peoples—such as "Hottentots" and "Australians"—held in the Paris Museum of Anthropology. The results were remarkable. The largest of all brains belonged, as was to be expected, to those who occupied the highest rung on the ladder of civilization—not just white men, but Parisian white men. (Ah, the French . . . you've gotta love them.) More surprising, though, was the ranking of civilized women, who came in below even the women of the most savage races: "In the most intelligent races, like the Parisians, there is a sizeable proportion of the female population whose skulls are closer in volume to those of gorillas than they are to the most developed male skulls." LeBon was swift to provide an explanation for this curious fact:

> In every human race, woman's skull is less voluminous than man's, but . . . the differences that exist between male and female skulls of the same race increase as one rises from the inferior to the superior races. . . . This . . . cannot surprise us. In inferior races, man's superiority over woman is minimal indeed. She shares his work, often even working harder than he does, and necessity makes her industrious. In completely civilised races, notably the Latin races, woman leads a very different life from man. The education she receives in no way exercises her intelligence and would tend to constrain rather than develop it. She thus remains stationary or regresses while, as man learns more and more with each generation, the cumulative progress of heredity ends up gradually distancing him more and more from woman from whom he was only very slightly distinguished intellectually in the beginning. . . . The races where male skulls occupy the top of the ladder are [thus] often precisely those where female skulls occupy the bottom rungs. . . . The skull of the female Parisian, indeed, ranks after the female skulls of inferior races where, obliged to share man's work, woman is forced to exercise her talents frequently.

It might sound like an argument for female education but, no, the reverse was the case. If civilized women were so much more stupid than civilized men, LeBon believed, it followed that this gap must be one of the markers of civilization and was to be messed with at society's peril.

> Those who have suggested giving women a similar education to that received by men have proved how little they understand her nature. . . . To give the two sexes, as they are starting to do in America, the same education, and by extension the same goals, is a dangerous chimaera that can only result in stripping woman of her role, forcing her to enter into competition with man, and taking from her everything that constitutes her value, usefulness and charm. The day when, holding in contempt the inferior occupations nature has given her, woman leaves her home and comes to share in our struggles, on that day will begin a social revolution that will see the disappearance of everything that today makes up the sacred bonds of the family, one that will be recognised in the future as the darkest of days.

THE SEARCH FOR DIFFERENCE

Attempts to find an explanation for differences between the sexes in the anatomy of the brain did not end with the nineteenth century. Although the gap in brain size between male and female humans is now considered to be simply a reflection of the two sexes' different body mass, the search for sex differences in the development, structure, and function of the brain is one of the liveliest areas of contemporary anatomical inquiry. The hunt is on for genes that might underlie such distinctions, with particular attention paid to those that live on the X and Y chromosomes. So far, there have been some interesting findings in fruit flies and nematodes, though any clear understanding of what different patterns of gene expression might mean for human males and females seems to be a way off.

When it comes to adult brains, the last ten to fifteen years have seen the identification of structural differences between the two sexes in every area of the brain, although some of these are small. The hippocampus, the area perhaps most associated with learning and memory, is said to be relatively larger in women than in men. Studies in rats and monkeys have shown chronic stress causes damage to this part of the brain in males but has much less, if any, impact in females. In contrast, the amygdala, the emotional center of the brain, is believed to be relatively bigger in men than in women.

Such research can be controversial, with some critics seeing it as representative of a "biological determinism" in the tradition of LeBon and friends. Differences in brain structure between men and women—and indeed between gay and straight people—have been promoted as explanations for a huge range of perceived behavioral, emotional, and cognitive differences. This is despite the fact that both the causes and effects of such anatomical variations remain largely mysterious to us.

Much of the research into sex differences in the brain has focused on the question of "laterality": that is, which side of the brain is more developed, or is used to complete a particular task, and how strong the connections between the two sides of the brain are. Because our brain is composed of two more or less symmetrical hemispheres, with each of its structures duplicated on each side (we talk about *the* amygdala, for example, but we actually have two of them), it is theoretically possible for us to complete the same task on either side or by using both in combination. It is often said that the left brain is the home of logical thought, while the right houses the emotions, as well as creativity and intuition. Although this distinction between the two hemispheres is by no means absolute, there are no prizes for guessing which sex is likely to be associated with each side.

Connecting the two hemispheres is a structure called the corpus callosum, a large bundle of nerve fibers that many researchers have claimed is larger in women than in men. This apparent greater connectivity between the two hemispheres in women has been suggested as an explanation for women's stronger verbal skills, intuitive nature, and greater ability to "multitask," as well as for men's mathematical and visuo-spatial skills and ability to focus more narrowly. Psychiatrist Robert Winston has even suggested it might underlie a male difficulty in expressing feelings, as men's emotional right brain would be unable to easily access the language centers housed on the left.

Not all scientists accept the ambitious claims made for the structural differences between male and female brains. Biologist Anne Fausto-Sterling, for example, questions, not just such interpretations but the very claim that the corpus callosum is bigger in women than in men. This connecting structure is so irregularly shaped and with so many of its nerve fibers protruding into, and becoming entangled with, other brain areas that it is impossible to measure accurately. It is, she says, "a pretty uncooperative medium for locating differences." In any case, she believes attempts to base theories about the psychology or cognitive abilities of the two sexes on such findings fail to acknowledge the complexity of the brain:

> The old-fashioned approach to understanding the brain was anatomical. Function could be located in particular parts of the brain. Ultimately function and anatomy were one. This idea underlies the corpus callosum debate. . . . Many scientists believe that a structural difference represents the brain location for measured behavioral differences. In contrast, connectionist models argue that function emerges from the complexity and strength of many neural connections acting at once. The system has some important characteristics: the responses are often nonlinear, the networks can be "trained" to respond in partic-

ular ways, the nature of the response is not easily predictable, and information is not located anywhere—rather, it is the net result of the many different connections and their differing strengths.

By allowing us to look inside the living brain, new imaging technologies are giving us a glimpse of that complexity. With functional magnetic resonance imaging (fMRI) and positron emission tomography (PET), researchers can watch the neurons fire as we complete a mathematical task, respond to a sexual stimulus, or recall the death of somebody we loved.

What such research is revealing is that there is no one way for the brain to carry out any particular task. Individuals can use various pathways and parts of the brain to achieve the same outcome, although many researchers do believe there are observable differences between men and women as groups. Functional differences between the sexes have now been described in fields as diverse as processing of emotion, memory, vision, hearing, face recognition, pain perception, navigation, and the action of stress hormones on the brain. Sometimes, the findings are linked to perceived behavioral differences between the sexes, but that is not always the case. Research suggests, for example, that the two sexes tend to use different regions of the brain to retrieve emotional, autobiographical memories, yet there is no difference in their ability to do this or in their level of emotional response. The sexes have also been found to perform equally well on an image naming task, but with significantly different patterns of brain activity.

Perhaps one of the qualities that most clearly distinguishes us from other animals is our sense of humor, and this too has become part of the hunt for differences between the sexes. Researchers at Stanford used fMRI to look at what was happening inside men and women's brains when they laughed at a joke. Men and women were asked to look at a series of cartoons and rate them for funniness. There was no difference in the number of cartoons the two sexes found funny or in how funny they found them. Both sexes responded equally quickly to the funny cartoons, though women were quicker than men to dismiss the unfunny ones. This behavioral similarity between the sexes was reflected in the activation of many of the same brain areas in both sexes, but there were some differences. Females activated areas of the left prefrontal cortex involved in executive processing and language decoding more than males, suggesting they might be using different strategies to respond to humor.

Although women did not rate the jokes as funnier than men did, the researchers were surprised to find amused females also showed more activity in the limbic system, the parts of the brain associated with "psychological reward." These are the areas that fire up when we win the lottery, look at a beautiful face, or take cocaine. The funnier the joke, the greater the difference in activity between the sexes in one small part of this system called the nucleus accumbens. But when a joke fell flat, the area barely responded in females while in males it was actually *deactivated.* Perhaps, the researchers suggested, this difference could be explained by differing expectations in men and women. Men were more likely to expect the joke to be funny, so their limbic system responded in surprise when it wasn't. Women were more pessimistic and thus had a greater response when a cartoon confounded their expectations by making them laugh.

Such questions are not of purely academic interest. Understanding sex differences in the brain's reward networks could lead to more targeted treatments for depression, which affects far more women than men (or at least is diagnosed more often in women), or addiction to computer games, which affects more men. More broadly, understanding of sex differences in the brain—if these were reliably established—could allow more effective treatment of men and women in conditions as varied as Alzheimer's disease, stroke, multiple sclerosis, schizophrenia, and attention deficit disorder.

Although they no longer claim women's brains are closer to gorillas' than to Parisian men's, researchers also still look to brain anatomy for clues to that vexed question of intelligence. There may be no evidence one sex is smarter than the other, but it has been suggested that various parts of the brain might make different contributions in men and in women.

Researchers at the University of California and the University of New Mexico used magnetic resonance imaging to examine the brains of men and women with equivalent IQ scores and found differences in the volume of white and grey matter in several brain regions. More grey matter in the frontal lobe was associated with greater intelligence in both sexes, but the other regions where volume of grey matter most strongly correlated with intelligence differed. For men, it was the parietal lobe, an area involved in space perception, movement, and touch. For women, it was Broca's area, one of the brain's language centers. It seems a sweet irony that the part of the brain named for the man who helped "prove" women were dumber than men is now believed to be larger and better developed in women.

The American researchers concluded: "Men and women apparently achieve similar IQ results with different brain regions, suggesting that there is no singular underlying neuroanatomical structure to general intelligence and that different types of brain designs may manifest equivalent intellectual performance."

Other research has indicated possible differences in how hard the brains of men and women have to work when completing various cognitive tasks. Male brains seem to be more neuronally efficient (that is, show less activation) when completing spatial cognitive tasks, while female brains seem to be more efficient at language-related tasks. This seems to fit with the general view that males have greater spatial abilities while females tend to be better at language, a difference often said to spring from our deep evolutionary past, when males supposedly needed better spatial skills to fulfill their role as "man the hunter." The observation of a difference, though, doesn't prove anything about its origins, evolutionary or otherwise, as we'll see later in this chapter.

Overall, a recent review of the neuroscience of intelligence concludes: "Apparently, males and females can achieve similar levels of overall intellectual performance by using differently structured brains in different ways." But the authors, from the University of Edinburgh, also point out that, although research tends to focus on differences between men and women, there are many reasons why individual brain function might vary apart from sex:

> Two individuals might achieve identical intelligence test scores through different neuronal routes because they have different brain structures or different expertise and training, or they might have used different cognitive strategies. . . . [There] seems to be substantial room for differences in how individuals use their brains for intelligent performance.

CHICKENS AND EGGS

We may be learning more every day about broad differences between male and female brains, but we are still a long way from understanding their causes or what such differences might mean for male and female *minds*— although that hasn't prevented construction of some elaborate theories of the gendered mind based on apparent biological differences.

Professor Simon Baron-Cohen is an English neurologist specializing in autism spectrum disorders including Asperger's syndrome, a group of conditions that are far more common in males than females. He believes these neurodevelopmental disorders, which involve impaired social and communication skills often in combination with narrow, obsessive interests and repetitive behaviors, can reveal general truths about male and female brains. Drawing on the work of Hans Asperger, who wrote in 1944 that the autistic personality was "an extreme variant of male intelligence," Baron-Cohen has elaborated an attention-grabbing and highly influential theory that

> the female brain is predominantly hard-wired for empathy. The male brain is predominantly hard-wired for understanding and building systems.

Although he is at pains to stress that these are average differences that will not apply to all individuals of either sex, Baron-Cohen suggests the brain is hard-wired by our genes and, in males, the consequent structuring role of testosterone. Here, Baron-Cohen strays into the realm of the evolutionary psychologist. Our most distant male ancestors might have evolved to become good systemizers, he suggests, because this improved their ability to make and use tools, hunt and track animals, trade goods, and negotiate power hierarchies. A lack of empathy might have helped them to dominate others, use aggression, and tolerate the solitude required to complete complex tasks.

On the female side of the equation, empathizing skills would have helped our ancestors to create group bonds and understand social dynamics, nurture children, and avoid male aggression. Although Baron-Cohen is unable to come up with an evolutionary advantage to be gained from poor systemizing skills in women, he suggests this lack probably wouldn't have caused any actual harm:

> that individual's superior empathizing could even have meant that when a system needed fixing (a tool was broken, a well had dried up), they had all the social skills to persuade a good systemizer to come and help them sort it out.

Baron-Cohen draws on research into cognitive and psychological differences between the sexes, studies of children's play and his own clinical experience with autism to bolster his theories. Perhaps the most striking piece of evidence is a study undertaken by two of his students who filmed more than a hundred one-day-old babies while they were shown two objects: a human face and a mechanical mobile. Analysis of the tapes showed the girls looked at the face for longer, while the boys spent more time looking at the mobile. This is a rare piece of evidence for very early sex-based differences (although it is often said that sex differences in the brain are "caused" by the action of testosterone in utero or immediately after birth, we actually have very little information about the structure of newborn human brains). That such a difference is present at birth strongly suggests biology is at work, Baron-Cohen concludes.

To assess whether individual adults have male or female brains, Baron-Cohen has designed two questionnaires to measure their Empathizing Quotient (EQ) and Systemizing Quotient (SQ). A high score for empathy and a low score for systems means a female brain, while the reverse indicates a male one. Similar scores on both reveal a "balanced brain."

There's an enjoyable navel-gazing element to doing quizzes like this, though it doesn't really feel like a very scientific exercise. It's easy enough to spot what the "right" answers would be if you happened to want a particular outcome. But that's not going to stop me and, I soon discover, has it stopped several of the female researchers I meet at an international autism conference a few days later. These scientific women seem quite chuffed at having come out with "male brains."

My own results are more ambiguous. I receive similar scores on both quotients, though slightly higher on empathizing than systemizing, which leaves me uncertain about whether I qualify as female or balanced. I also can't work out from Baron-Cohen's book what proportion of the population might be expected to fall into each of the categories he identifies. So I email him to ask. He obligingly responds by sending me one of his research papers on the topic. Plotting my scores on one of its graphs reveals I officially have a balanced brain, though tending toward the female side, but what surprises me is the answer to my second question.

The majority of women, according to Baron-Cohen's own figures, *do not have* a female brain. With 48.5 percent of women scoring female or extreme female, I'm left wondering in what sense something can be labeled "female" if it doesn't even apply to half of that sex. The remaining women are divided between balanced (35 percent of the total) and male (16.5 percent). Men do conform rather more to their expected gender profile with 59.6 percent scoring either male or extreme male, 23.7 percent balanced and 16.7 percent female.

Although Baron-Cohen's theories are intriguing, and the link with autism is particularly thought-provoking, I find myself wondering if seductively simple models of something as complex as the human brain are ever going to stand up to detailed scrutiny. I'm not the first one to have asked the question. Neuroscientist Lesley Rogers is a vehement critic of Baron-Cohen's work, arguing his belief in the hard-wired nature of sex differences leads him to underplay the role of the environment and learning. She cites research showing adults behave differently with babies depending on whether they are dressed as girls or boys as evidence of how early environmental influences can come into play. In a review of Baron-Cohen's book, she writes,

> I do not think there is anyone today who seriously contests that sex differences in brain function exist. What needs to be questioned is how large the average differences are and how meaningful they are in everyday life. Even more questionable are the assertions about ancestral humans, on whom natural selection is said to have acted to ensure that these differences became encoded in our genes. The main point that I want to make is that the existence of any average difference between the sexes tells us nothing about what causes them.

They're points that could as easily be made about many of the studies based on brain imaging. In most cases, we can only speculate about what causes the differences between male and female brains or about what their impact might be on behavior, cognitive style, or emotions. It's easy to think, and some of the neuroscientists seem to slide into this at times, that a difference in brain structure or function implies an "essential," pre-determined difference between the sexes. This plugs into the view that our biology is a given, a sort of primal layer on top of which environmental influences are overlaid. But such interpretations overlook the point made by Rogers and others about the constant interactions between biology and environment, with each influencing the other.

We know, for example, that environmental influences such as pollutants can affect the way genes are expressed in our bodies, and that our hormone levels fluctuate in response to stress. And nowhere is the influence of the environment on our biology more clearly seen than in the brain. The most plastic (that is, capable of change) organ in our body is constantly being shaped by our experiences, particularly those of early childhood when plasticity is at its greatest. What this means is that the more developed language centers in females, for example, could be as much a *result* of greater facility with language as they are the *cause* of it.

Studies suggest that women speak more fluently than men, remembering and using more words and organizing them into longer sentences. Males make more grammatical and pronunciation errors and are at least twice as likely to develop language disorders such as stuttering. In childhood, girls start talking about a month earlier than boys do and have bigger vocabularies and, from childhood to old age, females do better on tests of verbal memory than males.

So, is this an essential distinction between the sexes, programmed into our genes back in the hunter-gatherer days? Well, it could be. But it could just as easily be a learned difference. The saying "Use it or lose it" is particularly apt when it comes to the brain. The more we practice a particular function, the more established the neuronal pathways involved become and the easier and more automatic that task becomes. Another saying popular among neuroscientists is, "Neurons that fire together wire together." Just think about learning to drive a car. The first attempts can be terrifying (for both driver and passenger), with attention required to so many different inputs, and multiple tasks needing to be completed simultaneously. With practice, though, the whole thing becomes seamless and we often find ourselves doing it pretty much on auto-pilot. What we have done in learning such a complex task is actually rewire our brain, creating neuronal connections that will allow us to undertake it with a minimum of fuss. Research on people who have large parts of their brain wiped out by stroke is showing that even late in life we can train a different part of our brain to take over functions that were once performed in the damaged area.

Neuroscientist Walter Freeman has argued such plasticity is enhanced at crucial periods in our adult lives by the action of chemical substances in the brain, such as the so-called "feel-good hormone" oxytocin. This hormone is released in both sexes during orgasm, in parents when caring for their young children, and in children when they receive nurturing. It has also been called the "commitment hormone": in the monogamous prairie vole, levels of oxytocin (and a closely related male version called vasopressin) have been associated with greater fidelity between partners and bonding between parents of both sexes and offspring. At the autism conference I learn that an oxytocin nasal spray is being trialed as a possible treatment for that condition because of the hormone's role in enhancing perception of emotions and social behavior.

But oxytocin appears to do something else as well. Freeman suggests that it can actually encourage rewiring of the brain by erasing earlier pathways. What this means is that brain plasticity would be greater at those times that see large-scale release of the hormone: when we are starting a new relationship and when we have just become parents, for example. Falling in love, it seems, could actually trigger changes in our brain designed to enhance our compatibility with a new partner.

By far the most plastic period in brain development, though, occurs in early childhood, when our brains are required to absorb the enormous amounts of information we need to become functional members of human society. Although some degree of plasticity is retained throughout our lives, neuronal networks do become more fixed once the accelerated learning of childhood is complete. This is why we can learn to speak any language in the world as children but will find it difficult to achieve true fluency in a new language once we reach adulthood.

What all this means is that sex-based differences in adult brain structure cannot be separated from the experiences and learning an individual has been exposed to in childhood and beyond. If we foster language development more in girls than we do in boys, and girls then spend more time practicing their skills in this area, it would hardly be surprising if we found a structural impact in the brain. Baby girls may, in fact, be in linguistic training from birth, with research suggesting mothers spend more time talking to female infants than they do to male infants.

There is some evidence too that culture can affect the widely cited differences in cognitive abilities between the sexes. Although studies from many cultures do support greater male spatial ability, one 1960s study found the situation was reversed in the Inuit people of the Arctic where women's abilities were greater than men's. What's more, it is possible cognitive differences are on the wane in Western societies in response to cultural and educational shifts. A long-term analysis of scholastic aptitude tests in United States children found the expected sex differences were there for both verbal and spatial/mathematical skills but that they "declined precipitously" between 1947 and 1983.

Evidence such as this leads Lesley Rogers to conclude, "It is much easier to identify differences between the sexes than to find out what caused them. Part of the problem lies in the fact that, in all human societies, women and men have differences in both their biology and their social environments."

None of this is to say genetic and hormonal factors do not play a role in structuring the brain. We know genes from the X and Y chromosomes, including the male *SRY* gene, are active in various cells of the brain (although we don't yet know exactly what they do there). The brain is also populated with receptors that allow it to respond to the sex hormones.

But we also know that the brain more than any other organ in the body has the capacity to change in response to environmental influences. And we are increasingly coming to understand that even those biological factors, far from being fixed at birth, are subject to environmental influence. So, in a very real sense, it may be that we create our brains as much as they create us. Trying to pin down the relationship between "nature" and "nurture" is starting to feel like that old question of which came first, the chicken or the egg. The origins of any sex differences in the brain are too multifaceted for simple answers to be possible, Rogers tells me.

"There is no ultimate cause," she says. "And you don't need there to be."

Chapter Five

Learning Gender

In 1965, a pair of Winnipeg farm kids barely out of their teens became parents to twin baby boys named Bruce and Brian. One of those boys would become the central player in one of the most notorious, and tragic, cases in modern medicine.

At age eight months, Bruce was scheduled for a routine operation to relieve phimosis (an over-tight foreskin). Things went badly wrong. Using an electrocautery needle to remove the foreskin, the operating doctor accidentally burned off the little boy's entire penis.

What to do? Could a boy without a penis ever hope to become a happy, well-adjusted man? The family was referred to Johns Hopkins Hospital in Baltimore, home of one of the world's leading gender identity experts, psychologist John Money, who had considerable experience in working with children born with ambiguous genitals. Money believed intersex babies, and probably all newborn humans, were blank slates when it came to gender: "To use the Pygmalion allegory, one may begin with the same clay and fashion a god or a goddess," he wrote in 1972. The accidental removal of this baby boy's penis provided a rare opportunity for Money to test such theories in a non-intersex child, with, as an added bonus from a scientific point of view, a twin brother who could be used for comparison. Money recommended Bruce be raised as a girl and be given the surgery and hormonal treatment needed to support his new gender.

So Bruce became Brenda and, within a year of the original botched operation, had further surgery to, among other things, remove "her" testes. As the child grew, Money described her successful transformation in a series of publications using the pseudonyms "John" to describe the baby before the botched operation and "Joan" for the child after the gender reassignment. Nurture had conquered nature, with the new identity well accepted by both child and parents, Money wrote:

> Although the girl is not yet a woman, her record to date offers convincing evidence that the gender identity gate is open at birth for a normal child no less than for one born with unfinished sex organs or one who was prenatally over or underexposed to androgen, and that it stays open at least for something over a year after birth.

The "John/Joan" case was taken up by clinicians and gender theorists alike as evidence that gender roles were acquired rather than biologically determined. It was used to support the surgical approach to intersex children, the removal of male organs judged to be "inadequate" and the reassigning of such children as female.

It was only in the mid-1990s that cracks in the story began to appear. Psychologist Milton Diamond, a long-time opponent of Money's, and Keith Sigmundson, one of the psychiatrists who had treated Brenda as a teenager, wrote a paper revealing a far from happy history. They interviewed the adult Bruce, now living under the name David Reimer, as well as his wife and mother, and they reviewed Money's published accounts of the case. Reimer had decided he wanted his story made public to reduce the likelihood of others suffering as he had.

As a child, Brenda's behavior had occasionally been described as "feminine," the two authors found, but more often she was portrayed as a "tomboy," who preferred her brother's toys to her own and was more likely to imitate her father than her mother. Although she had never been told of her history, by around age ten a sense that she was not really a girl had begun to take shape. The adult Reimer remembered:

> There were little things from early on. I began to see how different I felt and was, from what I was supposed to be. But I didn't know what it meant. I thought I was a freak or something. . . . I looked at myself and said I don't like this type of clothing, I don't like the types of toys I was always being given. I like hanging around with the guys and climbing trees and stuff like that and girls don't like any of that stuff. I looked in the mirror and [saw] my shoulders [were] so wide. I mean there [was] nothing feminine about me . . . but I didn't want to admit it. I figured I didn't want to wind up opening a can of worms.

At age twelve, Brenda was started on estrogen supplements but often tried to dispose of them, saying they made her "feel funny." She was unhappy about the breast development they caused and refused to wear a bra. With no friends to support her—"Every day I was picked on, every day I was teased, every day I was threatened"—she had begun to have suicidal thoughts. When she was fourteen, other girls barred her from the female toilets at school, upset at her repeated attempts to urinate standing up. In the absence of a penis, the results were messy and her mother later recalled girls threatening to "kill" Brenda if she persisted.

At age fourteen, just before she reverted to the male sex, Brenda told her endocrinologist: "I suspected I was a boy since the second grade." Sigmundson and other local clinicians, who had observed the child's distress, oversaw the re-emergence of Bruce and the death of Brenda. Eventually, Bruce's father responded to prodding and, in a tearful episode, told his son the whole story. Bruce was relieved, though angry at having been lied to: "All of a sudden everything clicked. For the first time things made sense and I understood who and what I was," he later said.

He had his breasts surgically removed and started taking male hormones, to replace those that would have been produced by his testes if they had been left in place. While still a teenager, he had further surgical procedures in the attempt to construct a working penis, although this is a near-impossible thing to do. He ended up urinating through a fistula at the base of the constructed organ, which was largely without sensation as were the areas of scarring from which the required skin grafts had been taken.

Looking back, Reimer was scathing about the clinicians' focus on the penis as the be all and end all of male identity: "It dawned on me that these people gotta be pretty shallow if that's the only thing they think I've got going for me," he told Diamond and Sigmundson.

Although David Reimer did eventually marry and adopted his wife's children, this story does not have a happy ending. In 2004, he took a shotgun, sawed off the barrel, and shot himself in the parking lot of a local grocery store.

His biographer, John Colapinto, wrote that the real mystery was not why Reimer had committed suicide but how he had managed to stay alive for thirty-eight years, "given the physical and mental torments he suffered in childhood and that haunted him the rest of his life": "I'd argue that a less courageous person than David would have put an end to things long ago," he wrote.

This tragic case has been a political football in the gender arena for decades, with initial claims that it proved babies were a blank slate when it came to gender identity giving way to assertions that it instead proved gender was hard-wired from birth. But it seems to me the case never had the capacity to prove anything, except that the consequences of dogmatic beliefs in an area of such great uncertainty can be hair-raisingly cruel.

In no other area of science would a study of one individual be accepted as anything more than intriguing. Doctors would not be likely to base clinical decisions on a report that a single patient's asthma had improved after they took a particular drug, for example. To be truly meaningful, medical research requires an intervention to be tested in large populations and alongside controls who do not receive the treatment so that any placebo effect can be assessed. To eliminate the effects of observer bias, both participants and treating clinicians must remain unaware of who is getting the active treatment and who is receiving the placebo.

None of these requirements were met in the John/Joan case. Although Reimer himself was not told the story until age fourteen, his parents always knew their daughter had been born a boy. It would be silly to suggest they *could* have raised him in exactly the same way they would have raised a child who had been born female. In fact, throughout the twins' childhood this was a family in crisis. Colapinto reported that Brenda's guilt-ridden mother attempted suicide during this period, while her father "lapsed into mute alcoholism." As the family fell apart, the other twin, Brian, descended into drug use, petty crime, and clinical depression. Two years before Bruce's suicide, he died of a drug overdose.

I cannot agree with Diamond and Sigmundson when they conclude, "This update to a case originally accepted as a "classic" in fields ranging from medicine to the humanities completely reverses the conclusions and theory behind the original reports." It seems to me the sad outcome in the Reimer case *annihilates* those earlier conclusions, but that is not the same as reversing them. I find myself thinking that maybe there is yet another spectrum on which we all need to be measured: that of the rigidity of our gender identity.

In researching this book, I am discovering the myriad ways in which any individual can feel, understand, or project their gender. For some of the people I meet, gender is a fluid, ever-changing aspect of their identity, while for others (like, perhaps, David Reimer) it seems immutable from early childhood on. And, as we'll see in chapter 9, when we look at transsexualism, a rigidly held gender identity does not have to be one that matches a person's biology or appearance.

PLAYING WITH CARDS

When my daughter and son were small, I believed absolutely in the power of nurture over nature. I didn't quite dress them in the same clothes, but I gave them the same toys, read them the same stories, encouraged them to participate in the same mix of activities.

And, like many parents before and since, I ended up shaking my head in confusion at the results. Both of my children liked playing with cars, I used to tell my friends with a bewildered smile. But, when my daughter pushed a toy car across the floor, I would hear her saying: "Come on, darlings. We will get in the car and we will go to the shops and then we will go to visit our friends." In my son's case, the vocalizations pretty much consisted of "Brrrrrm. Crash. Brrrrrm. Crash."

Other parents reciprocated with laments that they had given their boys dolls only to see them decapitated or dismembered in various forms of rough play. Some sighed that banning toy guns was pointless as their sons turned every stick into a weapon they then pointed at their playmates to the accompaniment of machine gun noises. Most of the parental discomfort, and you could hear it from fathers as well as mothers, seemed to revolve around boys and what was seen as their more aggressive behavior.

Not all of my children's behavior was as stereotypical as the car play might suggest, but still I found it confusing because I could not remember ever having enacted such stereotypes in my own childhood. For a girl growing up in the 1960s and 1970s, I was fortunate in having remarkably few of them imposed on me. It's true I was occasionally forced into a dress when visiting the grandparents, but nobody ever made me think there was anything wrong with the fact that I preferred climbing trees to playing with dolls. Many, perhaps most, of my women friends had similarly boisterous childhoods. We were, I suppose, what some people would call "tomboys," though I have always disliked the term, preferring to see an active, outdoorsy childhood as just one of many possible ways of being a girl rather than some sort of pseudo-maleness. It's not as though my identity as a female was ever in doubt, although my amused mother did find me standing on the toilet seat at the age of five in an attempt to pee standing up like my friend Peter from across the road.

My ideological commitment to nurture over nature bit the dust a long time ago, as simple ideologies will tend to do in the face of the complex realities of parenting. My children grew into the adults they were going to be, with their own idiosyncratic mix of qualities, some typical of their respective genders, some not. But I have often wondered where that stereotypical behavior of early childhood came from, what function it played in the formation of their identities.

Psychology researchers, I discover, have grappled with the same question. Children, they say, already have some awareness of gender stereotypes by age three, including ideas about appearance, dress, and toys—girls wear dresses, boys play with cars. Their knowledge of stereotypes expands rapidly over the next three years, encompassing more abstract concepts such as jobs and personalities—men drive trucks, women are "nice." As is the way with children, these little gender policemen and women can be put out when people fail to fit the classifications they have learned. Other children who engage in cross-gender behavior are particularly frowned upon and can be mercilessly teased. It certainly rings a bell with me when I read that children's gender stereotypes are at their most rigid, in relation to both their own and others' behavior, around the time they start primary school.

"Stereotypes are likely to be held quite rigidly until [about age eight] as younger children do not seem to recognize that there can be individual variation in masculinity and femininity within the male and female categories," the authors of a review wrote.

One researcher recorded this exchange between an aide and a four-and-a-half-year-old boy who was trying to unfasten the clasp of a necklace in a preschool playground:

Aide: Do you want to put that on?

Boy: No. It's for girls.

Aide: You don't have to be a girl to wear things around your neck. Kings wear things around their necks. You could pretend you're a king.

Boy: I'm not a king. I'm a boy.

Children's knowledge of gender stereotypes seems to keep growing throughout their primary school years, but they become less likely to see them as inflexible or "morally" right. It seems the stereotypes impose more of a straitjacket on boys than they do on girls, however: "girls are both more knowledgeable and, after the preschool years, more flexible in their personal acceptance of gender stereotypes, and boys hold stereotypic views more rigidly and are held to them more by others."

It's hardly surprising then that many studies suggest boys become more and more likely to stick to gender-typed activities as they move through primary school, while girls if anything go in the other direction.

The embracing of gender stereotypes seems to be a key way that children learn their own and others' gender. As any parent knows, children love consistency and predictability. It's a big, confusing world out there and they're going to hang on to any certainties they can find. That's one reason why they make us play the same game over and over, and read the same story till we feel like taking out a contract on the very hungry caterpillar. They need to know that the story will *always* end in the same way, that Daddy will *always* come back when he plays peek-a-boo. Maybe learning, and enacting, the rules of gender operates in a similar way.

The search for scientific order could start here, with the small child's need to impose predictable patterns on something as inherently slippery and hard to grasp as sex and gender.

JOHN IS A BOY, BETTY IS A GIRL

Psychological theories of gender development have to grapple with complex, overlapping inputs. There's the question of how much a sense of gender might be innate, programmed into us by genes and hormones and just waiting to be "discovered" by our developing minds. Then there's the input of parents and other caregivers, the ways we learn our gender by observing and imitating them or from their rewarding or punitive responses to our own behavior. Peers have an influence too: we want to be accepted by our tribe, whether that is boys or girls. And then there's the bombardment of messages from society and the media about what is and is not appropriate behavior for somebody born with our particular brand of biology.

The various theoretical approaches give different weightings to each of these inputs, but what we do know from psychological research is that gender makes its presence felt early. Research suggests we treat boys and girls differently from babyhood on, even when their behavior is exactly the same. One study, for example, found adults saw babies as stronger and less sensitive when told they were male, regardless of the babies' actual sex. Other studies suggest mothers smile more at their infant daughters than they do at sons and that both mothers and fathers show more physical affection to girls than to boys. Babies themselves become aware of gender early. Seven-month-olds respond differently to male and female voices and, by age one, many also show different responses to male and female faces.

By two and a half, most toddlers are using gender-specific words like "he" and "she." Children, especially boys, are more likely to play with toys conventionally associated with their gender (dolls for girls, cars for boys) and both boys and girls are starting to show some preference for playing with other members of the same sex. Around three, children seem to grasp the idea that gender is a fixed aspect of people's identity, something that will not change just because they put on different clothes or engage in different activities.

The condition clinicians call "gender identity disorder" (which we'll come back to in chapter 9) can make its first appearance during these preschool years. The causes of this mismatch between anatomy and identity remain mysterious, but small children with a persistent desire to belong to the other sex may refuse to wear clothes or engage in activities generally associated with their own biological sex. They may also show revulsion for their genitals, trying to hide them or imitate those of the other sex. For some of these children, the discomfort with their gender will pass, while others will go on to become transsexual adults. It's a curious fact that girls are more

likely than boys to express a desire to belong to the other sex during childhood, although adult transsexualism is far more common in the other direction.

Some researchers have speculated that little boys have traditionally
needed to engage in a more active rejection of femininity because so many of
the important adults in their lives have been female. Although fathers are
much more involved in caring for their young children today than they were
a few generations ago, boys still tend to spend more time with women than
they do with men. Preschools, child care centers, and even primary schools
are predominantly staffed by women. Because both sexes construct their
gender through a combination of imitating others of the same sex and differ-
entiating themselves from those of the other sex, boys who do not spend
much time with male role models may have to rely more on the second. They
may in effect define their gender not as "like" men but as "different from"
women. Psychologist Leslie Brody writes,

> Without an available male role model, boys cannot imitate their fathers' emo-
> tional expressiveness, but rather, are theorized to develop a masculine gender
> identity by becoming different from their mothers in emotional expressive-
> ness . . . [leading to] minimization of emotional expression, especially in a
> social context in which expressing intense emotions is considered to be "femi-
> nine."

We know that girls are more likely to imitate a male role model than boys are
a female one, although boys will sometimes break this taboo if the female is
seen as exceptionally powerful. Perhaps it's not surprising that fathers have
more success than mothers do in persuading children, especially boys, to
engage in activities normally associated with the other sex.

The peer group can reinforce stereotypical behaviors, Brody writes, with
research showing boys who "conform to masculine display rules are viewed
as 'cool.'" Conforming means not showing feelings of rejection or vulner-
ability:

> Popular boys also act "tough" and aggressive, challenge adult authority, and
> boast and brag about their sometimes rule-violating exploits. . . . Boys who are
> low in popularity are those who are seen as vulnerable or weak, who cry
> easily, or who are the most frequently hurt or defeated in athletic games, the
> so-called "sissies."

In contrast, popular girls are those who are good at verbal expression, who
understand group dynamics, are less aggressive, and are interested in social
relationships.

Children's plastic brains are quick to respond to such social norms, to observe and reproduce the behaviors that are rewarded or punished in each sex in their particular culture. The responses of parents, other caregivers, and their peers all tell them how they should behave if they wish to gain the rewards of approval, love, and friendship. Perhaps the most striking of these is that old chestnut, "Big boys don't cry," which for all the changes in gender roles in our society can still be heard in every playground when a little boy falls and grazes his knee. Little girls it seems are allowed to cry but, for the boy, his status as both male and "not a baby" is under threat if he allows himself the release of tears.

As I read the psychological research, I find myself wondering why we are so *hard* on little boys, why we won't let them cry, why we are so punitive when they behave in a way we associate with the other sex. It's not the first time I've had such thoughts. Back when my children were enacting gender stereotypes in their play with cars, I was doing graduate study in psychoanalytic theory. Although, like most people these days, I was more amused than convinced by Freud's famous arguments about the role penis envy and castration anxiety played in girls' and boys' formation of gender identity, I found some of the post-Freudian work on male identity formation intriguing. Psychoanalyst Robert Stoller, for example, wrote,

> [T]he whole process of becoming masculine is at risk in the little boy from the day of birth on; his still-to-be-created masculinity is endangered by the primary, profound, primeval oneness with mother, a blissful experience that serves, buried but active in the core of one's identity, as a focus which, throughout life, can attract one to regress back to that primitive oneness. That is the threat latent in masculinity.

It seems almost like a psychological version of the biological process described in chapter 1. Children start off psychologically "female," because of their early unity with the mother, and masculinity can only be achieved by an active overcoming, indeed a rejection, of that primal femaleness. The results of this arduous process can be harsh, especially for those little boys who do not easily fit into the stereotypical male mold, and I find myself wondering if (hoping, even) men's increased involvement in caring for their young children might not be doing something to relax such pressures.

Even with the dramatic shifts we have seen in gender roles over recent decades, though, children are still bombarded with subtle, and not so subtle, messages about how each sex behaves. They may notice that their father generally drives the car whenever both parents are present, or that their primary school teacher always asks boys to help when she needs to move a table. Parental arguments may end in maternal tears and a paternal disappearance. Or their grandfather may always put out a hand to steady their grandmother when she goes to cross the road.

And, of course, all of this happens within a broader social context. No matter what gender values parents portray to their children, we are all subject to the imagery of a larger, and increasingly visual, world. Let's think for a minute about the messages each sex receives about itself.

A little girl growing up in an affluent Western household will be bombarded with images of the female through the media, consumer objects, educational materials, and public spaces. The women she sees in public forums, such as television news, will tend to be younger than the men, perhaps less authoritative, certainly more sexualized. Advertising is filled with images of near-naked women, often accompanied by star-struck men. She may play with Bratz dolls, or something like them, plastic pre-teens with pouting lips, revealing clothes, and big, flirtatious eyes. She and her peers sport modified versions of this adult wear: crop tops and empty bikini tops. At her birthday party, a friend may give her a toy make-up set or offer to paint her toenails. This is not the entire picture, of course, but it is a large part of it.

What does this girl's brother see? Men in public forums are more likely to occupy positions of authority or to be the attention-seeking clown (often with a woman playing straight guy). Men are also more likely to be the bad guys. When a footballer is involved in a sex scandal or a businessman in corporate fraud, this too sends a message to the small boy. In advertising, however, men are often shown as rather stupid, even infantilized, with perhaps a more competent woman taking charge to fix the problems they have created. The message our little boy is likely to get is that men are more powerful and attention-seeking than women, but that they are also a bit hopeless when it comes to managing the practicalities of life. Men, it seems, continue to need a mother all their lives.

Perhaps more profoundly, much of the imagery around gender reinforces the binary. Male and female characters tend to be placed together but in opposition. The man is often drably dressed, while the woman is colorful. If he is loud, she is quiet. If he is stupid, she is smart. If he is good, she is bad. And so on. The qualities ascribed to each sex can be reversed, but the binary is maintained. If there is one clear message our little girl and boy receive, it is that there are two categories of people in the world and they are fundamentally different from each other.

THE TWO TRIBES

The primary school playgrounds of my childhood had a white line painted down the middle separating the boys from the girls. The idea behind this appeared to be that boys were in some way inherently *dangerous* and girls needed to be protected from them. Teachers patrolled the white line to enforce border control, though there were many male incursions into the forbidden female territory. The most daring was the time a group of boys managed to scramble to the top of the walls of the unroofed female toilet block so that they could look down at the little girls peeing below.

It's hard to imagine a Western school enforcing such segregation today, but research suggests children left to their own devices will create their own white lines on the tarmac. In the psychological literature, primary school children are often portrayed as two separate tribes or cultures, segregated by sex, with male groups based around "rough and tumble play" and competitive dominance hierarchies while female groups are seen as more verbal and co-operative (a view that might be challenged by many women who have survived such groups!). This sex segregation has been described as a "powerful developmental phenomenon that increases with age and potentially serves as a mechanism for socializing children into the ways of their own gender group."

Children who try to break out of this gender apartheid to play with the other sex can have a hard time of it. As I am working on this book, a boy I know is grappling with just such a problem. Although "rough play" comes in at number three on his list of favorite things in the world (after drawing and reading, but ahead of computer and television), he has always enjoyed the company of girls and boys equally. When he was younger this wasn't a problem but, at seven, he is being teased by other boys, and the girls, while happy to keep playing with him at home, have started excluding him from their group play at school.

Research shows a large minority of primary school children do engage in some behaviors considered atypical for their gender (23 percent of boys, 39 percent of girls) but, once again, rebellion is harder for boys. They are likely to be teased, shunned, or referred to as "girls" if they don't stick with their tribe and comply with stereotypes about how boys behave.

The funny thing is that, although children hold strong stereotypes about how boys and girls behave, studies tend to show the actual differences in their behavior are not that great. Girls, for example, are generally considered more helpful than boys, but research finds only small and inconsistent differences in behavior. Similarly, girls are perceived as more passive and dependent but research into their behavior does not support this. And while girls *say* they feel more empathy for others, observational studies do not find any difference between the sexes.

Studies have, however, found some emotional differences between the sexes, increasingly so as they get older. While there are few differences between babies and toddlers, by early primary school, boys are more likely to hide feelings of sadness and girls are less likely to express anger. By adolescence, girls report greater intensity of emotions and more sadness, shame, and guilt, while boys are more likely to deny such feelings.

Psychologist Janet Shibley Hyde argues the traditional research focus on differences between the sexes, and the huge popular interest in the subject, may have actually obscured the very substantial similarities between males and females. She outlines a "gender similarities hypothesis" arguing that men and women, and boys and girls, are similar "on most, but not all, psychological variables." Her statistical approach finds that most observed differences between the sexes actually belong in the "close to zero" or small range, with only a few in the moderate range and very few classified as large or very large.

Among the 78 percent of differences Hyde found to be small or close to zero were qualities or behaviors often strongly associated with females (communication, self-disclosure, ability to process facial expressions, and helpfulness) and others believed to be stronger in males (leadership, activeness, interrupting, and most math skills). Males were moderately more likely to show aggression, with the evidence stronger for physical than verbal aggression. The evidence that females engaged in more relational aggression (such as excluding one child from play) was ambiguous, Hyde found. There was one area where large differences were found between the sexes (guess who's more likely to masturbate), but we'll come back to that in chapter 7.

One of the problems with many psychological studies, as Hyde and others have pointed out, is that they tend to look at people outside their social context and can thus under- or overestimate behaviors. Studies of aggression, for example, generally do not find major differences between men and women, yet we assume there is a real-world difference given the evidence that men are far more likely to commit violent crimes.

To see boys and girls developing in their social context, we need to turn to the social sciences. Barrie Thorne is an ethnographer who set out to study sex segregation in American primary schools. Initially, he found himself focusing on situations that epitomized the separation between boys and girls (a game of chase between gangs of boys and girls in the playground, a classroom math game that saw the teacher organize the class into "Beastly Boys" and "Gossipy Girls").

But then Thorne began to realize he was overlooking as "less interesting" a host of more positive and cooperative interactions between the sexes. Gender segregation was not absolute, he found. Three boys and two girls joined up in the classroom to produce and record a radio play. One girl in a fourth and fifth grade composite class regularly hung out with the popular, sporty group of boys. Spanish-speaking kids of both sexes, excluded from other play by a lack of English, played dodge ball together in the playground. And, outside the conformist world of the primary school, in families and neighbor-hoods, children were even more likely to play with the other sex because "there are fewer witnesses to tease girls and boys who choose to be together."

Most of the research on children and gender involves a search for individ-ual or group differences, the magnitude of which is often exaggerated, thus reinforcing the sense of the sexes as opposites, Thorne writes. In the process, real-world complexity is obscured:

> In everyday life in schools, children and adults talk about the different "na-tures" of girls and boys primarily to justify exclusion or separation and in situations of gender conflict. . . . [Such] moments seem to express core truths: that boys and girls are separate and fundamentally different as individuals and as groups. They help sustain a sense of dualism in the face of enormous variation and complex circumstances. But the complexities are also part of the story. In daily school life many situations are organized along lines other than gender, and girls and boys interact in relaxed and non-gender-marked ways.

Conventional literature on sex-role socialization paints children as passive recipients of gender identities, Thorne says, rather than seeing them as active participants who construct and resist culture as well as adapting to dominant ideologies.

Educational sociologist Diane Reay is one researcher who has examined the cultures primary school children create through a study of the ways seven-year-olds in an inner London primary school performed their gender. Although her study mostly focused on the girls' various group cultures, she also recorded this exchange between two boys who took turns interviewing each other, each making an endearing attempt to imitate the style of an adult interviewer:

Josh: David, what do you like most about being a boy?

David: Well, it must be that it's much easier to do things than being a girl, that's what I think. You get to do much better things.

Josh: So you think you find being a boy more interesting than being a girl? Is that what you're saying?

David: Yes, because it's boring being a girl.

Josh: OK, and what do you like least about being a boy?

David: Well, I don't know, I can't think of anything.

Josh: Well, can't you think really—there must be something.

David: I'll think [long pause]. Well, it's easier to hurt yourself.

Then it's David's turn to ask the questions.

David: OK, what do you like most about being a boy?

Josh: I'd probably say that it's better being a boy because they have more interesting things to do and it's more exciting for them in life I find.

David: Yes, I see. What do you like least about being a boy?

Josh: Ohh, I'd probably say not being so attractive as girls probably I'd say they're much more attractive than boys.

Interestingly, Reay describes both boys as popular with peers (perhaps because they were perceived as "clever"), despite their not entirely conforming to the dominant ideas about masculinity in their working-class school. David, in particular, was studious and hated games when the dominant interest of the other boys was playing or talking about football.

When it came to the girls in the class, Reay divided them into four overlapping and largely self-defined groups. There were the "nice girls" who were hard working and well behaved, the ultra-feminine "girlies" who wrote love letters and flirted with the largely uninterested boys, the more assertively pre-sexual "spice girls" and the "tomboys." Both of the first two groups tended to be looked down on by the boys and the other girls. The boys described the girlies as "stupid" and "dumb" (despite the fact that their educational performance tended to be better than the boys'). In one group discussion, three of the other girls agreed that "no one wants to be a nice girl." Other children described the nice girls as "boring" or "not fun" and the boys saw them as contagious and polluting. Not surprisingly, the nice girls themselves saw it differently. Here's an exchange between two of them:

Emma: The other girls often mess around and be silly; that's why Alice and Lisa never get their work finished.

Donna: Yes, we're more sensible than they are.

Emma: And cleverer.

Like the girlies, the spice girls engaged in a lot of pre-sexual behavior like flirting and bemoaning their broken hearts, but they were more assertive about it. A favorite playground game was "rating"—they would follow boys around and give them a mark out of ten for attractiveness. Two of these girls got into trouble for forcing David's hand into a bowl of treacle during a science class to punish him for "showing off [and] making out he knows all the answers." The incident made David cry and convinced the class teacher the two girls were "a bad lot." Teachers responded more harshly to such bullying behavior when it was carried out by girls than by boys, Reay found.

Of all the groups, Reay found the tomboys the most intriguing. One of these girls, Jodie, said, "Girls are crap, all the girls in this class act all stupid and girlie." This did not include her, she said, because she was, "not a girl. I'm a tomboy." She had no female friends because girls did not share her interests, particularly football. Well, some of them *liked* it, "but they're no good at it." Reay saw Jodie's rejection of a feminine role as cementing rather than transforming the gender divide. In her field notes, she found sixteen examples of Jodie asserting that "boys are better than girls." The diversity of gender roles enacted in this class led Reay to conclude that performing gender was not straightforward. In fact, it was downright confusing:

> The seduction of binaries such as male:female, boy:girl often prevents us from seeing the full range of diversity and differentiation existing within one gender as well as between categories of male and female.

Chapter Six

The Third and Many Genders

One of anthropology's favorite parlor games is the search for universals, the attributes that can be found in all human societies and can therefore be considered an intrinsic part of what it means to be human. Inspired by linguist Noam Chomsky's *Universal Grammar*, anthropologist Donald Brown has collected hundreds of them: we use language to mislead, we gossip, we're scared of snakes, we dance, we dream, we envy, we measure, we suck our thumbs, we marry, we style our hair, we try to predict the future, we fear death, and we tickle.

Among the universals are a number of qualities that relate to our need to order and categorize the world (making a list of human universals in itself would have to be a demonstration of that). The tendency to organize knowledge into binary categories is on the list, as is the distinction we draw between culture and nature. And a host of entries start with the words "classification of" followed by subjects as varied as age, behavioral propensities, body parts, inner states, kin, and, of course, sex. In every culture, sex and gender terminology is fundamentally binary, and males and females are seen as having different natures, Brown says.

Unsurprisingly, sex, gender, and sexuality crop up repeatedly on the list. All societies are said to have division of labor by sex, with males dominating the public or political realm, while females do more direct child care. Men on average travel greater distances over the course of a lifetime and there are sex differences in spatial cognition. We impose regulations on sexuality, particularly to prevent incest, and we generally have sex in private. Males are more aggressive, more violent, and more likely to steal. Rape occurs in every society but is also universally proscribed. And women usually have a consort during their child-rearing years, with husbands on average being older than wives.

You could argue about many of the things Brown includes on his list, particularly perhaps about his contention that every culture views sex in binary terms. Nigerian anthropologist Oyeronke Oyewumi has, for example, criticized her Western colleagues for imposing on other, non-Western, cultures their view of gender as *the* organizing principle of the social world. In her own analysis of West Africa's Yoruba people, she finds individuals are defined more by age than sex. This is reflected in the language: Yoruba pronouns do not indicate sex (there is no he or she), but rather the relative ages of the people involved (something like "older one," "younger one"). Perhaps even more problematic for the assumption of a universal sex binary is the existence in some cultures of what is sometimes called a "third sex," a gender category that is neither male nor female, something we'll come back to later in this chapter.

Some might argue about the validity of even attempting to define universal qualities of human beings, given the potential such a project has to obscure the enormous differences between cultures. But Brown's list has a certain charm and it does raise interesting questions about what it means to be human. I find it hard to resist the idea of defining humanity as the species that tickles.

SEX AT WORK

If human cultures have generally allocated labor roles according to sex, the question I want to ask is *why*. In most societies, sex-based division of labor is much more far-reaching than you might expect if it was based simply on physical differences between the sexes, such as men's greater strength or women's reproductive role. Wouldn't basing allocation of tasks on individual talent or interest be more productive? The Western world does, in fact, seem to have moved in that direction, making it increasingly hard to maintain the claim that a sex-based division of labor roles exists in every society. After all, if anthropology is going to make claims about universals, it's going to need to be able to apply them to our urbanized Western societies as much as to people living in the remote highlands of Papua New Guinea. Although many work roles in contemporary societies are still dominated by one sex or the other, I can't think of a job that is *never* performed by the non-typical sex (though I have to admit I don't remember ever seeing a woman hanging off the back of a garbage truck). Some anthropologists have also pointed out that labor roles are not strictly adhered to in every non-Western society, as we'll see with the Agta people of the Philippines.

Still, for most of human history, biological sex does seem to have been an organizing principle, perhaps *the* organizing principle, for dividing up the work that needed to be done. An explanation might be found in the fact that, to avoid in-breeding, human societies tend to marry out. One sex, most often the female, will leave its community of origin to find a marriage partner elsewhere. Communities who swap their young women in this way need to know the newcomers will have the same skills as those who left. You wouldn't want to send away all your weavers, only to get a pack of hunters in return. So it makes sense to standardize the skills taught to individuals of each sex across tribes or villages. Incidentally, this practice of women marrying out is also sometimes seen as underlying the supposed female advantage in communication and personal skills, necessary tools for survival if you are dumped into a strange community.

In some societies, the tasks allocated to the two sexes can seem pretty arbitrary. In one place, pottery may be the province of men, in another of women. But others are, if not exactly universal, more common across cultures. Men's greater strength makes them more likely to take on roles such as fighting and hunting, for example, although women are known to have done some hunting in many cultures, from the Tiwi people of the islands off northern Australia to the nomadic Plains tribes of North America (not to mention the odd U.S. vice presidential candidate). Male dominance in hunting and fighting extends into other related areas that do not in themselves require any particular physical strength, such as weapon making. The argument seems reasonably plausible, though it's worth noting that carrying heavy loads such as water and firewood, which also requires physical strength, has tended to be a female responsibility and remains so in much of the developing world today.

The physical constraints imposed on women by their role in reproducing the species are also often seen as underlying universal differences. Pregnancy and lactation restrict women's mobility, the argument goes, limiting their access to activities such as hunting or long-distance trading and making them more suited to occupations such as cooking and working with textiles. This has led to a common definition of man's sphere as "public," while woman's is "domestic."

I can't help feeling we're heading back into evolutionary psychology territory here—the shadow of Man the Hunter looms large—and a number of anthropologists have in fact argued that the sharp distinction between these two spheres is a hangover from a nineteenth-century world view. "Many of us have tired of the domestic-public dichotomy. We feel that it is constraining, a trap," writes anthropologist Louise Lamphere. It certainly seems an inadequate model outside the industrialized world, where the two spheres are hard to distinguish. The more I read of such material, the more circular the argument comes to seem: when a woman does something, it is defined as domestic; when a man undertakes the same task, it is more likely to be seen as public. If a woman grows food for her family and sells some of her produce at market, for example, which is that? And what of a man teaching his son how to make a household implement? This account of seventeenth- and eighteenth-century Iroquois society shows the difficulty of drawing a clear line between the two worlds:

> Iroquois matrons preserved, stored, and dispensed the corn, meat, fish, berries, squashes and fats that were buried in special pits or kept in the long house. . . . [W]omen's control over the dispensation of the foods they produced, and meat as well, gave them de facto power to veto declarations of war and to intervene to bring about peace. . . . Women also guarded the "tribal public treasure" kept in the long house, the wampum quill and feather work, and furs.

Although the actual roles given to the sexes may vary, male roles do tend to be valued more highly. As pioneering anthropologist Margaret Mead wrote in the 1940s:

> In every known society, the male's need for achievement can be recognized. Men may cook, or weave, or dress dolls or hunt hummingbirds, but if such activities are appropriate occupations of men, then the whole society, men and women alike, votes them as important. When the same occupations are per- formed by women, they are regarded as less important.

There are cultures, though, where individuals can take on some or all of the tasks of the other sex without apparent censure. Often, this requires them to take on a different gender identity, becoming seen as a member of the other sex—or of a "third sex" as we'll see further on in this chapter. But some cultures have allowed their members to do the work of the other sex without this affecting identity. Among the nomadic Plains cultures of North America, women could at times participate in traditionally male occupations such as hunting and warfare without losing their status as women. A "manly hearted" woman might, for example, join a male war party to exact retribution for the death of a relative.

Perhaps the most striking example of a culture where gender roles are not rigidly enforced is that of the Agta people who inhabit the mountainous region of the Sierra Madre in the northeastern Philippines, a society under pressure from population influxes and deforestation. Anthropologists Agnes Estioko-Griffin and P. Bion Griffin spent several years in the 1980s living among the Agta and found both sexes crossed boundaries when it came to gender roles. Men, for example, were observed helping with work normally done by women, such as tying fronds to the roof of a shelter or the laborious process of extracting flour starch from the caryota palm.

And Agta women could be enthusiastic and skillful hunters. Members of communities closer to lowland Filipino settlements laughed when asked about female hunters, saying such things would only happen among the wild, uncivilized people living deep in the mountains, but the Griffins went on to encounter groups where hunting was a common occupation for both sexes. While still young, girls and boys were taught forest knowledge, starting to hunt animals such as wild pig, deer, or monkey from puberty and continuing into old age. Hunting parties, armed with dogs and machetes or bows and arrows, could be all-male, all-female, or mixed: a woman might hunt with her husband or with her brothers, sisters, or other relatives. Women were less active hunters while their children were small, although other family members, including occasionally fathers, would sometimes care for children to let them have a go.

When it came to sexual relationships, the Griffins found that polygamy was not common among the Agta, but they documented several cases of polygyny and one rare instance of polyandry—a woman with two husbands, one older, one younger. The other women apparently found this arrangement amusing but acceptable, though when the Griffins described it to an old man in a settlement further to the south, he was less tolerant. "Well, perhaps one man with two wives is OK," he said, after pausing to digest the information. "But a woman with two husbands? I find that totally bad." The surrounding women, the Griffins recorded, just laughed at him.

MAKING MEN

Among the Masai and other cattle-herding tribes of East Africa, young boys are taken from their mothers around the time of puberty and subjected to bloody circumcision rites designed to turn them into men. Anthropologist David Gilmore writes,

> They must submit without so much as flinching under the agony of the knife. If a boy cries out while his flesh is being cut, if he so much as blinks an eye or turns his head, he is shamed for life as unworthy of manhood, and his entire lineage is shamed as a nursery of weaklings. After this very public ordeal, the young initiates are isolated in special dormitories in the wilderness. There, thrust on their own devices, they learn the tasks of a responsible manhood: cattle rustling, raiding, killing, survival in the bush. If their long apprenticeship is successful, they return to society as men and are only then permitted to take a wife.

Although they are not always as harsh as the Masai, societies around the globe routinely require young males to "prove" their manhood, often through tests of strength or courage. Gilmore's roll call of manhood rituals includes the beating and terrorizing of boys in the New Guinea highlands, the sheep stealing and competitive game playing of Crete, the requirement that an African !Kung boy single-handedly track and kill an adult antelope, the merciless whipping of boys from the Tewa people of New Mexico by "spirits" who are really their fathers in disguise, and the English upper classes' relinquishing of their sons to the vicious world of the public boarding school.

Why, Gilmore asks, do so many cultures enact such harsh manhood rituals, when they do not require equivalent trials from girls on the verge of womanhood? Across cultures, manhood is seen as something that has to be *achieved*, rather than just an inevitable consequence of biological maleness. Although women may be judged when they behave in socially unacceptable ways, it is rare for their identity *as women* to come into question, he argues. Yet manhood is seen as precarious, something boys must win against powerful odds:

> True manhood is a precious and elusive status beyond mere maleness . . . [that] frequently shows an inner insecurity that needs dramatic proof. Its vindication is doubtful, resting on rigid codes of decisive action in many spheres of life: as husband, father, lover, provider, warrior. A restricted status, there are always men who fail the test.

The first thought that comes into my mind reading this is that the female sex would be unlikely to feel a need to *invent* complicated trials by ordeal since biology has given us our own violent testing ground in the form of childbirth. Western women these days may be able to choose not to put themselves through it, but for most women throughout history giving birth has been central to their status within family and community. If we want torture, we don't need to go off into the forest to find it. The labor ward of our local hospital will do.

Gilmore does not discuss the role childbirth might play in achieving womanhood, but he does come up with another explanation for the omnipresent rituals of manhood, one that echoes some of the psychological theories discussed in the last chapter. Small boys, he argues, face a special burden and peril that their sisters are spared because they must escape their early bond with their mother if they are to achieve an independent, masculine identity:

> To become a separate person the boy must perform a great deed. He must pass a test; he must break the chain to his mother. He must renounce his bond to her and seek his own way in the world. His masculinity thus represents his separation from his mother and his entry into a new and independent social status recognized as distinct and opposite from hers.

THE THIRD SEX

Clinicians who work with transsexual or intersex people often speak wistfully of countries like Thailand where, they say, there is a place for people whose psychology or anatomy places them outside the gender binary. The "lady boys" of that country occupy a space between male and female that is widely accepted by their compatriots, I'm told. And, in fact, while I'm researching my article on children with non-standard gender identities, photos of a high school in northern Thailand appear on the Internet, or rather photos of the school's toilet block adorned with a stylized half-male, half-female sign. According to media reports, androgynous students at this Chiang Mai school were unwelcome in the girls' toilets but refused to use the boys', forcing authorities to provide a third option.

The question of toilets always seems to come up when you start talking about ambiguities of sex or gender. For transsexual people, there's often a quandary about when exactly during the transition process they should start using the unaccustomed conveniences of their new sex: do they look male enough, or female enough, to pass without comment? But the issue seems to make everybody anxious, not just those who have to make an active decision about which door they go through. The choice of toilets is an early and public marker of gender, its importance magnified by the association with shameful bodily functions.

I've been wondering if the Thais are really as accepting of gender ambiguity as everybody says, so when, on a trip to Brisbane, I get chatting to two young flight attendants from Thai Airways who are on a layover in the city, I take the opportunity to ask their views. Kamnan is shy and conservatively dressed, her friend Kitti more the extrovert in tiny little shorts, high-heeled ankle boots, teased hair, and lots of bling. Kamnan and Kitti (not their real names) tell me they hate flying to the Gulf, where the women are covered up and the men stare at them. As we eat Japanese food together, I tell them about my book and that I have heard they have high schools with three toilets in Thailand.

"*One* high school," Kamnan says sternly.

Are people accepting of such things, I ask, and she screws up her face in distaste: "Not everybody is liking this."

Peter Jackson is a specialist in Thai history who has extensively researched the country's gender and sexual identities and confirms that Westerners sometimes take a rose-colored view of supposed Thai liberalism. He writes,

> Western observers, including many foreign gay visitors, commonly view Thai culture as expressing liberal, even accepting, attitudes towards male transgenderism (*kathoey*) and masculine-identified male homosexuality (gay). . . . Idyl-

lic accounts of Thailand as a "gay paradise" are at odds with anti-homosexual views that have long been expressed in both popular and official discourses, which are often stridently critical and intolerant of non-normative sex/gender behaviors.

He is not the only one to caution against Western appropriation of gender identities in other cultures to suit our own arguments and needs. Academic Susan Stryker, herself a transgender woman, writes of the uneasy fascination Westerners have felt for exotic configurations of gender and the way this has become entwined with our perceptions of other, colonized races:

> For half a millenium now, Eurocentric culture has been treated to a parade of gender exotics, culled from native cultures around the world: Indian *hijra*, Polynesian *mahu*, Thai *kathoey*, Brazilian *travesti*, Arabian *xanith*, Native American *berdache*—and so on. "Transgenders," at home and abroad, are the latest specimens added to the menagerie.

Even with such cautions in mind, it does however seem that some of those cultures Stryker mentions have found a place for people who do not neatly fit the gender binary in a way we in the West have struggled to do.

Anthropologist Gilbert Herdt describes Indian society, for example, as "highly gender-polarized between men and women," but he also sees it as including one of the world's most significant examples of a third sex. The ascetic caste of the hijra is composed of men who dress as women after undergoing voluntary (and, these days, illegal) castration. The hijras worship the mother goddess and have a special place in religious rituals such as blessing marriages and births. Anthropologist Serena Nanda has written about the ambiguous position hijras hold in Indian society:

> The hijras, as human beings who are neither man nor woman, call into question the basic social categories of gender on which Indian society is built. This makes the hijras objects of fear, abuse, ridicule, and sometimes pity. But hijras . . . are also conceptualized as special, sacred beings, through a ritual transformation . . . sexually ambiguous figures are associated with sexual specializations; in myth and through ritual, such figures become powerful symbols of the divine and of generativity.

As members of an ascetic caste, hijras are supposed to be celibate but many are sexually active and some even work as prostitutes.

Some of the most striking examples of a third sex, to me at least, are to be found in the Americas. Early in that half-millenium-long history of European fascination with exotic genders, explorer Pedro de Magalhaes de Gandavo in 1576 described the Tupinamba people of northern Brazil:

There are some Indian women who determine to remain chaste: these have no commerce with men in any manner, nor would they consent to it if refusal meant death. They give up all the duties of women and imitate men, and follow men's pursuits as if they were not women. They wear the hair cut in the same way as the men, and go to war with bows and arrows and pursue game, always in company with men; each has a woman to serve her, to whom she says she is married, and they treat each other and speak with each other as man and wife.

I can't help suspecting "chaste" is not the most accurate word to describe the lives of these women.

In North America, examples of "two-spirit" people have been documented in more than a hundred indigenous tribes, in many of which they apparently enjoyed high status or were considered to have special powers. Personal inclination seems to have played an important part in setting somebody on this life path, with cross-gender behaviors in childhood often seen as indicating the future role.

Some two-spirit people took their identification to extremes. Among the Mohave, such men would enact female roles, including scratching their inner thighs till they bled to simulate menstruation and eating plants that caused constipation so that they could experience something approximating the exertions of childbirth.

Most accounts of a third sex describe men taking on a female identity, something that has provoked debate among anthropologists. I find myself wondering if this, and the fact that male-to-female transsexualism is more common in the West than is the reverse, might be related to the more rigid gender roles so often demanded of men. There can be many ways to be a woman but manhood, as we have seen, may be much less accommodating of variety.

Nonetheless, many North American tribes did include women who took on a male role. Among the Mohave again, *hwame* girls were said to reject the female role because they had dreamed they would be boys while still in the womb. If adults failed to discourage them from their chosen path, these children would go through a special ritual that authorized them to take on a male identity, including marrying a woman. This didn't mean they were entirely accepted as men, however, as wives of hwame could be teased about their "inadequate" husbands.

In the frozen north of the continent, where people relied on male hunting to survive, female children were sometimes designated male for economic reasons. It seems unlikely the individual child had much choice in the matter, making it perhaps a cruel life. Among the Kaska people of the sub-Arctic, a couple who had too many daughters would simply select one of them to "be like a man." From about age five, such a child was required always to wear a belt adorned with the dried ovaries of a bear, believed to prevent menstruation and pregnancy and bring good luck on the hunt. She was dressed like a male and trained to do male tasks. As adults, these women had female sexual partners and would react violently if a man made sexual advances to them because, as Kaska people explained: "She knows that if he gets her then her luck with game will be broken."

A recurrent theme in these third sex roles from different continents is the blurring of two categories we in the West have only recently begun to separate: gender identity and sexual orientation. Homosexuality in our cultures too has often been portrayed as a kind of intermediate gender, with gay men stereotypically seen as "effeminate" and lesbians as "butch." Similarly, in the early days of transsexual surgery, sexual orientation was one of the criteria for gaining approval for the procedure. A biological male seeking surgical realignment as a woman was *expected* to want penetrative sex with a man. The pioneer of the medical treatment of transsexualism, Harry Benjamin, in 1954 wrote,

> Homosexual inclinations always exist in the transsexualist whether they result in actual physical contacts or not. . . . The interpretation of the libido as homosexual is strongly rejected by the male transsexualists. They consider the fact that they are attracted to men natural because they feel as women and consider themselves of the female sex. For them to be attracted to "other females" appears to be a perversion.

Benjamin is still admired by many in the transsexual community for his pioneering role in declaring the condition could not be "cured" psychologically and was best treated with hormones and possibly surgery. But his conviction that all transsexual people shared the same sexual orientation has been shown to be laughably wrong as we'll see in later chapters.

Clinicians no longer see a particular sexual orientation as a criterion for sex-change surgery, but homosexuality is still often portrayed as a kind of intermediate gender in Western scientific literature. Some studies purport to show that "gay brains" are similar to those of the other sex, while other research suggests children with gender identity issues are more likely than others to be gay in adulthood.

Outside the world of science, distinctions between gender identity and sexual orientation are not always clear-cut either. Gay people more often than straight people take a playful approach to gender, breaking down distinctions through drag or by consciously taking on behaviors normally associated with the other sex. With increasing acceptance and visibility of homosexuality, such practices have had an influence on all of us, contributing to a more flexible attitude to gender in Western societies. We in the West may not have an institutionalized third sex, as some cultures do, but we are more tolerant than we used to be of people who blur the boundaries.

Chapter Seven

Sexing Sexuality

It should be superfluous to caution the readers of this book against becoming familiar with girls or women who are entire strangers, and taking personal liberties with them. A young man takes the step immediately leading to this great peril when he invites a girl, with or without a hint from her, to an unchaperoned automobile pleasure ride. Ordinarily the very acceptance of such a ride stamps a girl as being without honor, self-respect and shame. Her company is disgraceful, and association with her is perilous morally, physically, socially and financially. Not seldom the leprosy of her diseased body is as contagious and deadly as is the lechery of her degraded soul. Many an unsophisticated and adventurous young man has been completely ruined for life by one such injudicious and deadly ride.
(*Safeguards of Chastity*, 1929)

My grandmother, Freda, would have been twenty-one years old and the proud owner of her own automobile when the Franciscan friar, Fulgence Mayer, published his advice about the dangers of such vehicles. I am sure Freda never used the car she inherited from a fond uncle to lead young men astray but she did, many years later, want to pass on some of the lessons learned in her own youth to my daughter, her great-granddaughter. Watch out, she said, for boys who bring an attaché case on a date. Confused, we asked what would be in the case? A *picnic rug*, she replied ominously.

The instruments of seduction are many and Friar Fulgence struggled to come up with effective strategies to help young men avoid them. "It is by no means easy for a young man to be and stay chaste," he wrote. Apart from avoiding leprous females in cars, regular bowel movements and a hobby might help. But the detailed advice he offered on how to confess the sin if a young man lapsed suggested he was perhaps not all that optimistic. The multiple choice template reads in part: "I have sinned by impure thoughts about once or twice, or oftener, a week, or a day; by impure desires . . . feelings . . . looks . . . touches . . . with myself . . . with girls . . . with boys . . . with close relatives . . . with animals."

Friar Fulgence probably battled against the idea, but for most of us our sexuality, and the body that expresses it, is a central part of our identity as a human being. It's hardly surprising that scientists, philosophers, and theologians have long debated the nature of this urge, with a particular focus on its manifestations in the two sexes. Which sex is the more libidinous is a perennial subject of interest. The authors of the 1486 anti-witchcraft tract, the *Malleus Maleficarum* (Hammer of Witches), wrote that woman was a "wheedling and secret" enemy:

> All witchcraft comes from carnal lust, which is in women insatiable. . . . [T]hree general vices appear to have special dominion over wicked women, namely, infidelity, ambition, and lust. . . . [S]ince of these three vices the last chiefly predominates, women being insatiable, etc., it follows that those among ambitious women are more deeply infected who are more hot to satisfy their filthy lusts; and such are adulteresses, fornicatresses, and the concubines of the Great.

In the more sedate Victorian era, British gynecologist William Acton wrote in 1857 that, "the majority of women (happily for society) are not very much troubled with sexual feeling of any kind."

These days, neither sex is seen as exactly "untroubled," although both science and popular culture are more likely to portray the male of the species as the insatiable one. When psychologist Janet Shibley Hyde outlined the gender similarities hypothesis (see chapter 5 of this book), she argued almost all psychological differences between the sexes were in the close to zero or small range. The one big exception was in sexual behaviors and attitudes. Although there was almost no difference in reported sexual satisfaction between the sexes, the same could not be said for other markers, she wrote. "Gender differences are strikingly large for incidences of masturbation and for attitudes about sex in a casual, uncommitted relationship."

How do you quantify something as slippery and indefinable as desire? The authors of one recent review of the psychological research decided it was necessary to look at a whole lot of different measures if they wanted to determine which sex had the stronger sex drive, and they were adamant about the results:

> By all measures, men have a stronger sex drive than women. Men think about sex more often, experience more frequent sexual arousal, have more frequent and varied fantasies, desire sex more often, desire more partners, masturbate more, want sex sooner, are less able or willing to live without sexual gratification, initiate more and refuse less sex, desire and enjoy a broader range of

sexual practices, have more favorable and permissive attitudes toward most
sexual activities, have fewer complaints about low sex drive in themselves (but
more about their partners), and rate their sex drives as stronger than women.
There were no measures that showed women having stronger drives than men.

Although women had a greater *capacity* for sex—they could perform the act
more often, with more partners, and could have more orgasms—they had on
average less desire for it, the researchers wrote, arguing the difference between the sexes was most likely caused by a combination of biology (principally, testosterone) and cultural influences.

One of the places these researchers sought evidence of a fundamental
difference between the sexes was in the sexual behavior of gay men and
lesbians. In that never-ending (and probably futile) search for the "natural"
behavior of men and women, they are not the first to have sought in homosexuality a picture of male and female desire unconstrained by the need to
compromise with the other sex. Gay men, the argument often goes, behave as
all men would if they could get away with it. And lesbians act as all women
would if they didn't have to worry about men. Hence the joke that two gay
men will, within five minutes of meeting each other, be trying to set up a
threesome, while two lesbians will be looking at moving in together and
getting a cat.

There are, of course, plenty of raunchy lesbians out there—as a few
minutes on YouTube will demonstrate. But the learned Dr. Acton would
probably have concurred with such a denial of female desire (always assum-
ing he could have been convinced of the existence of such a thing as a
homosexual female). I do have to wonder about the assumptions behind such
analyses, especially the apparent belief that gay sexuality is somehow more
representative of "natural" human behavior than anybody else's. None of us
escapes the influence of the wider culture or the subcultures that may be
associated with our particular brand of sexuality.

Still, even to the outside observer, there do seem to be some pretty obvious differences between male and female homosexual behavior, and studies
show gay men have more frequent sex and many more sexual partners than
do lesbians. In the course of researching this book, I met somebody who is in
the unusual position of having been an insider in the gay cultures of *both*
sexes. Born female, this trans man was a lesbian until he decided to transition
to a male identity in his early twenties, at which point he found himself
feeling attracted to men for the first time. While he remains with his female
partner, he also has casual relationships with gay men. Online dating sites
used by the two groups are radically different, he says,

On the lesbian versions, the photos will be of them with their dog, or babies, or their best friend, and it's all about, "These are my favorite authors, la, la, la, la . . ." And on the boys' sites, it's, "Here's a photo of my cock. Here's what I like. Here's what you need to be like. I'm cut/I'm not cut. I engage in these activities . . ." Like, everything . . . well it works, for its purpose.

Another gay man with a transsexual history is even more expressive. When he first entered the gay scene, he wondered if he would be able to find partners, given that he didn't have a penis and had still not had chest surgery to remove his breasts, but his fears proved unfounded. "Honestly, some men will go for anything," he says. "They are so indiscriminate, seriously, they will do a watermelon."

It's hard to dispute the existence of differences between the sexes when it comes to sexuality, but there are some clues that the size of those differences may have been exaggerated. Research in this area always relies on what men and women *say* they get up to. And they might be telling the truth.

Or they might not.

In fact, we know somebody's lying on at least one of the measures often used in research. When it comes to the average number of heterosexual partners men and women have, the number across the whole population has to be the same. But it isn't. In multiple studies, men on average report having had significantly more heterosexual partners than women do. Unless large numbers of extraterrestrial females are involved, this is a mathematical impossibility. Either men are exaggerating the number of partners they have had, or women are under-estimating, or both.

Other studies have found men consistently claim to have heterosexual encounters more often than women do, another statistical impossibility. Less clear-cut, but also suspicious, is the fact that straight men claim on average to have lost their virginity at a younger age than women. For this to be true, older girls would need to be making a practice of having sex with younger boys. It's possible, but it certainly doesn't gel with my observations or experience of adolescence.

So, if we know people are prepared to lie to researchers about some aspects of their sexual behavior, it seems reasonable to suspect they might also lie in response to other questions, such as those about masturbation, fantasies, or specific practices they have engaged in. Although social attitudes to sexuality in the West have changed dramatically over the last half-century, expectations about appropriate behaviors are still not identical for the two sexes. A large 2007 study found the double standard was alive and well in college students across the United States, for example. Women who had a lot of casual sexual encounters were described as "sluts" by both sexes, whereas men who behaved in the same way were often admired by male peers for their frequency of "scoring." Men were also more likely than women to say they respected somebody less for agreeing to such an encounter and tended to see women who abstained as better relationship material.

Even allowing for the fact that Americans are probably more conservative than other Westerners when it comes to sex, such attitudes help explain why men might be tempted to err on the side of generosity when describing their sexual achievements, while women might be shy about acknowledging the extent of theirs. My instinctive response was to put the discrepancies down to male boasting, but it seems possible it is actually the women who are the dissemblers.

American psychologists asked two hundred straight, single college students a series of questions about their sexual history and attitudes, with the aim of working out how honestly each sex responded and how real the reported differences in sexual behavior between the sexes were. One group was led to believe their written answers might be seen by another student working as a research assistant, the second was promised their responses would be strictly anonymous, and the third was told they were hooked up to a lie detector while they were filling out the forms. (The lie detector actually wasn't operational, but participants didn't know that.) The researchers believed the students would be most truthful when connected to the lie detector and least when they thought their responses might be read by another student.

Sure enough, the biggest differences between the sexes' description of their own sexual behavior were found when people believed the experimenter would be able to view their answers. When participants believed they could be caught out by the lie detector, differences between the sexes were negligible. Although men in all groups reported more masturbation and use of pornography, the gap between the sexes was significantly smaller in the anonymous and lie-detector groups, suggesting women might feel embarrassed about admitting to such practices.

When it came to that vexed issue of numbers of sexual partners, once again it looked as though it was the women rather than the men who were reluctant to tell the truth. Although the findings did not reach statistical significance, the trend is certainly intriguing. The biggest sex difference in reported numbers of partners was found in the group who believed their responses might not be private: an average of 3.7 partners for the men, compared with 2.6 for the women. The gap was smaller in the anonymous group, at 4.2 for men and 3.4 for women. And, in the lie-detector group, it was actually reversed, with women reporting an average 4.4 partners and men 4.

Interestingly, these researchers found the overall differences in responses between the men and women were "not particularly robust," echoing other recent research suggesting the gap between the sexes on sexual attitudes and behaviors might be narrowing in Western cultures. "As a given society advances toward gender equality," they wrote, "differences in gender role expectations may diminish, rendering sex differences in self-reports of sexuality obsolete."

Researchers who conducted a global study of sexual attitudes and behaviors did not go so far as suggesting the differences between the sexes might become obsolete—in fact, they said they found moderate to large differences across cultures and argued this supported the evolutionary psychology perspective that links sexual behavior to parental investment strategies (see chapter 2). But they also found women's "sociosexuality"—a term used to describe a spectrum of mating strategies from monogamy to promiscuity—became more like men's when society treated the two sexes more equally. "When progressive sex roles give them the opportunity, it appears, both men and women tend toward sexually promiscuous attitudes and behaviors," they wrote.

An earlier American study had found 22 percent of men raised before the sexual revolution of the 1960s (and the advent of reliable contraception) had five or more partners before age twenty, compared with only 1 percent of women. For those who came of age during the 1960s, however, the figures were 30 percent for men and 11.5 percent for women—that's around a 1,000 percent increase for women within the space of a few years. Women were also more likely to be sexually adventurous in wealthy societies where resources were plentiful and lives were long, but adopted a more conservative approach in more precarious environments, the authors of the global study found. They concluded,

> Women never precisely match the sociosexual psychology of men, but women's overall level of sociosexuality comes closer to men's when it is given the chance. The current findings support the view that women's sexuality is often constrained by cultural values and social institutions, and the "true" nature of women's sexuality includes short-term mating desires and some degree of sexual promiscuity.

THE ELUSIVE ORGASM

"A brief episode of physical release from the vasocongestion and myotonic increment developed in response to sexual stimuli," was how pioneering sex researchers William Masters and Virginia Johnson described the orgasm in 1966. I doubt many people would consider that an adequate representation of the experience, but then the sensation is notoriously difficult to capture in words (although D. H. Lawrence certainly tried).

Researchers in the 1970s asked male and female college students to describe their orgasms in an attempt to assess whether there was any difference in the sexes' subjective experience of the phenomenon. The descriptions were certainly more evocative than that of Masters and Johnson. For example,

> Basically it's an enormous buildup of tension, anxiety, strain followed by a period of total oblivion to sensation then a tremendous expulsion of the buildup with a feeling of wonderfulness and relief.

> A sudden feeling of lightheadedness followed by an intense feeling of relief and elation. A rush. Intense muscular spasms of the whole body. Sense of euphoria followed by deep peace and relaxation.

> Feels like tension building up till you think it can't build up any more, then release. The orgasm is both the highest point of tension and the release almost at the same time.

The students' accounts, with any gender-specific anatomical details removed, were shown to a group of male and female experts—doctors, psychologists, and medical students—to see if they could work out which ones described a male orgasm and which ones a female. They couldn't.

If the sensation of orgasm is similar in the two sexes, so too is the physiological process of arousal and satisfaction. Male or female, our hearts beat faster, we breathe more quickly and shallowly, and blood rushes to our genitals causing our penis, or clitoris and labia, to swell. If the engorged areas receive the right stimulation for the right amount of time, our brains and genitals will cooperate to produce the rhythmic contractions and pleasurable sensations of climax. Females can stay aroused after a first orgasm and keep repeating the experience, while in males the climax will usually, though not always, be accompanied by ejaculation and detumescence.

The pioneer of sexual research and family planning, Marie Stopes, early last century wrote that men could practice birth control by training themselves not to ejaculate during sex. The key apparently was to focus on "the spiritual aspect of the beloved," though Stopes herself was not convinced: "In my opinion an average, strong and unimaginative Englishman is not likely to achieve success in this type of union, but more sensitive and artistic temperaments and those in which the vitality is not excessive undoubtedly can do so."

When it comes to understanding what actually happens when we have an orgasm, science still has a lot to learn. Despite the best efforts of Masters and Johnson, and earlier of Alfred Kinsey, studying the sex act in humans has always had a whiff of the disreputable about it. And there are inevitable questions about how well sex under laboratory conditions replicates the experiences most of us have in private.

You might think it happens between your legs, but actually "experiencing orgasm is a function of the brain," say researchers at the University of Groningen in the Netherlands who have been doing their best to overcome the research difficulties. Despite the rapid advances in imaging technology in recent years, looking inside the brain during sexual activity is no easy task. Quality images require the body part under consideration to remain still, clearly a challenge in the case of sexual intercourse. The Dutch researchers have had to fall back on studying orgasms produced through manual stimulation by a partner. During this process, participants' heads are immobilized to facilitate the PET scan of their brain and a rectal probe is inserted to monitor pelvic contractions and verify reported orgasms have actually occurred. That all twelve women in one study managed to have an orgasm—not to mention that four of them came twice and two of them three times—seems to speak to the power of human desire. Or maybe the setting was more erotic than it sounds.

There was considerable overlap in the orgasmic brains of men and women, although there were also some differences, the researchers found. There was more activation of parts of the brain involved in sensations of touch in men than in women. In both sexes, but especially in women, brain regions associated with behavioral control showed reduced activity during orgasm. Research leader Gert Holstege told the London *Times* this suggested "letting go of all fear and anxiety might be the most important thing, even necessary, to have an orgasm."

Females are both more and less orgasmic than males: climax is harder to achieve but they can also come repeatedly within a short space of time. Reliable figures are hard to get, but it's estimated that 10 to 20 percent of women may have serious difficulty reaching a climax. Men, of course, have their own sexual difficulties, especially as they age, but being unable to reach orgasm during penetrative sex is not usually one of them.

Stopes was ahead of her time when she started campaigning for recognition of the female orgasm, even going so far as to provide a detailed description of the clitoris. Much of the neuroticism of early twentieth-century women could be attributed to the fact they were aroused in the marital bed and then left unsatisfied, she believed. In her 1918 book, *Married Love*, she advised doctors to question any woman with sleeping problems about whether her husband "really fulfils his marital duty in their physical relation." The multiple editions of her books indicate she certainly found an audience, but I wonder how many medical practitioners heeded her advice. Stopes herself disapprovingly quoted a "distinguished American doctor" who in 1900 wrote, "I do not believe mutual pleasure in the sexual act has any particular bearing on the happiness of life."

The 2007 study of casual sexual encounters among American college students indicates such attitudes may not have entirely disappeared. Women in this study were far less likely than their male companions to reach orgasm, partly, it appeared, because of a greater focus on male satisfaction in the encounters. In couples who did not have penetrative sex, for example, the men were three times more likely than the women to be the only ones to receive oral sex. Some men admitted that, if they saw the encounter as a one-off, they didn't much care about the woman's orgasm. "I mean like if you're just like hooking up with someone, I guess it's more of a selfish thing," said one. In other cases, the men did try but were unsure of just how to get there. And others were deceived by women faking it. Women said they did this to make the man feel good, "to make them feel like they've done their job," or "just really to end it."

I can't help feeling a bit sorry for those boys saying they *tried* but they didn't really know how to make sure their partner had an orgasm. Where once the emphasis was all on restraint, these days it sometimes seems to be all about performance. Are you a good kisser? Do you give good head? How many orgasms do you have or give? One man earnestly tells me that he likes watching porn because it gives him ideas and I can't repress an unfortunate image of him, notebook in hand, formulating programs for future sexual encounters. For men, the number of orgasms a woman has can be a measure of their prowess, which I suppose is why some women end up faking it.

It's hard to believe that science not that long ago was still questioning the very existence of the female orgasm. When Kinsey revealed in the 1950s that 14 percent of American women reported, not just having them, but having them in multiples, the suggestion was ridiculed by rival experts. Psychoanalyst Edmund Berger and gynecologist William Kroger declared, "One of the most fantastic tales female volunteers told Kinsey (who believed it) was that of multiple orgasm. The 14 percent belonged obviously to the nymphomaniac type of frigidity where excitement mounts repeatedly without reaching a climax. Kinsey was taken in by the near-misses."

Of course he was. Although the existence of the female orgasm, even in multiple form, is no longer controversial, scientists still shake their heads over *why* such an apparently useless phenomenon would have come into being. It (and the clitoris) have even been compared to male nipples, a vestigial remnant of something necessary in one sex that persists for no apparent reason in the other. It never seems to occur to the people who make such arguments that, if the female orgasm is not essential for purposes of reproduction, than neither is the male. Male *ejaculation* is necessary for conception to occur, but there is no biological reason why it has to be accompanied by the pleasurable sensations of orgasm.

Various evolutionary explanations for the female orgasm have, in fact, been proposed, most commonly that the accompanying contractions might help to keep sperm in the vagina and propel them toward the cervix. Even the capricious nature of the female orgasm could be an evolutionary adaptation, it has been suggested. If a woman has several partners during her fertile period, this might mean the one who brings her to climax has a better chance of getting to fertilize the egg. The evidence linking orgasm to increased likelihood of conception is not conclusive, but it seems to me there could be a much simpler explanation. Women would probably be more inclined to mate with those men who gave them orgasms and, more generally, making the sex act pleasurable for both participants would have to help promote the reproduction of the species.

LAWS OF ATTRACTION

Desire is one of the things that define us as human beings: that unpredictable, indefinable force that takes hold of us, enhancing sensation and dulling judgment. Why we feel it for some people and not for others tends to be mysterious to us. Men and women can often be heard puzzling about the apparent lack of pattern in their former partners. And how is it we can be entranced with desire for one person at first meeting, while another apparently more suitable candidate leaves us cold?

The evolutionary psychologists seek answers in our drive to access the best genes for our future progeny, which makes some sense. Such forces operate even when we have no intention of reproducing, or so the argument goes. Facial and bodily symmetry, and other markers of good health, tell us a potential mate will contribute to quality offspring. Both sexes emit pheromones, sending olfactory signals about their reproductive fitness and genetic make-up. Women may emit signals around the time of ovulation to let men know they are at their most fertile and they also seem to be better able to smell male pheromones at this time.

Evolutionary impulses are not limited to our unconscious evaluation of the health of a prospective partner's genes. We also want to know what sort of parent they might make. A study that sought to establish the kinds of faces we find most attractive found some surprising results. Researchers digitally manipulated photos of men and women to produce a series of images from most "feminized" to most "masculinized." Then they asked people in two very different cultures, Japan and Scotland, to rate the faces for attractiveness. It was no surprise that respondents in both countries preferred women with more feminine faces, but the researchers were taken aback to find people also found the feminized men more attractive than the average or masculine ones. The masculine faces were seen as more dominant, cold, and dishonest, and as less cooperative and less likely to make good parents.

A follow-up study further complicated the picture. Women, it turned out, were attracted to different types of men depending on the stage of their menstrual cycle. Around the time of ovulation, they were more likely to opt for the masculine faces, suggesting they might favor the more co-operative, feminized men as long-term partners but take the opportunity to access some more macho genes when they were at their most fertile.

"As in some other species, selection might have favoured human females who pursued a mixed mating strategy," the authors wrote. "A female might choose a primary partner whose low masculine appearance suggests co-operation in parental care ('long-term' preferences are unchanged across the menstrual cycle) but occasionally copulate with a male with a more masculine appearance (indicating good immunocompetence) when conception is more likely."

Other studies have suggested men and women look for different things in a mate, with men tending to focus on youth, fertility, and the attributes of a good homemaker, while women tend to look for an older man who is a good provider. Cross-cultural research has shown that such preferences are less marked in more egalitarian societies where labor roles for the two sexes are similar, although the evidence from online dating sites seems to support the enduring power of some of the stereotypes. One recent study of twenty-two thousand heterosexual users in Boston and San Diego looked at the volume of contacts men and women received, rather than what people *said* they were looking for, to evaluate the qualities perceived as most attractive by the other sex. Physical attractiveness was important to both sexes, but women preferred older, taller, slightly overweight men, while men went for younger, shorter, underweight women. Men's success increased substantially with their income, but this had no impact for women. Men also didn't care about women's occupations, but women did care about men's with the most popular jobs being, in order, lawyers, firefighters, soldiers, and the health professions.

Although evolutionary explanations for some of these mate preferences have a certain plausibility, they struggle to come to grips with the diversity of human desire. As Friar Fulgence noticed in his cautionary advice to young men, our sex drive can have many objects, not all of them linked to a reproductive outcome. We can be attracted to people of the same sex, to those we know to be infertile, even to inanimate objects. The enterprising and bisexual Dr. Kinsey apparently explored the parameters of his own desire by filming himself masturbating with a swizzle stick up his urethra. For some people, sexual desire can even become focused on a directly anti-reproductive practice such as castration performed as an erotic act.

How we develop our sexual orientation, and why it turns in a particular direction, is still largely a mystery. Researchers have sought various biological explanations for homosexuality, even occasionally announcing the discovery of a "gay gene." (It always puzzles me that nobody ever talks about the hunt for the "straight gene"—you'd think, if one type of sexual preference could be ruled by something as simple as a single gene, they all could.)

My hunch is that, like so many other attributes of us humans, our sexual orientation is far too complex to be ruled by one gene, or even a bunch of genes acting in concert. It is probably formed by ongoing interactions between our biology and environment, with each influencing the other in ways unique to each individual. Orientation can form early, even before the time when we might think of ourselves as becoming sexual beings: one study of young gay and bi men found they were aware of being attracted to other males before age ten. I'm not sure you could productively ask that question of a straight person. I have no idea when I first knew I was attracted to males, probably because belonging to the dominant majority meant I felt no need to question my orientation.

It's interesting to wonder how many of us might have had the capacity to go in more than one direction if circumstances had been different. One scientist tells me he thinks most of us probably have some degree of attraction for both sexes, with only a small number at either end of the spectrum absolutely hetero or homosexual. (And some theorists would question even the existence of such categories since they rely on accepting the binary nature of sex.) Certainly, a lot of "straight" people have had a homosexual experience at some point in their lives, without it necessarily affecting how they see their identity, and I wouldn't be the first to observe a homoerotic element in a lot of male team sports. In fact, while I'm working on this book, I'm told about a Sydney brothel that experiences a surge in allegedly straight male customers requesting anal penetration on nights following a big rugby league game.

Some researchers suggest female sexuality is more plastic (that is, changeable) than male in relation to various factors including orientation, although homosexuality is generally considered to be less common in women than in men. Gay and straight women are more likely to be aroused by both male and female sexual stimuli, whereas male arousal is more tightly linked to sexual orientation. Another study found a quarter of eighteen to twenty-five-year-old women who identified as lesbian or bisexual changed their orientation over a five-year period. Such an identity shift was less common in men. It sounds like the joke about women being "lesbian till graduation" and it might indicate a greater female willingness to experiment. I can't help suspecting, though, that homoerotic practices (communal masturbation, for example) are more common in adolescent boys than in girls and that perhaps the difference is more about how people define their identities than about actual sexual practices.

On the face of it, the prevalence of homosexuality across human cultures would seem to go against arguments for a dominant evolutionary role in mate selection. While I can't see any need to find an evolutionary explanation for homosexuality, given how often our human sexual practices are removed from a reproductive role, I can think of one reason why those hypothetical "gay genes" might have prospered. Parenting is not the only way we can further the survival of our genetic material. Our children may carry 50 percent of our genes on into a new generation, but our nieces and nephews will also carry 25 percent of them. Children with devoted, and childless, aunts and uncles might well stand a better chance of survival. Having a strain of homosexuality in the family could offer an evolutionary advantage.

Chapter Eight

Testosterone and Friends

Aram has been through puberty twice—the first time as a female, the second as a male. When he decided to transition from a female to a male identity at the age of twenty-three, he started having regular injections of testosterone to masculinize his body. And the surge of hormones plunged him into all the turmoil of a male adolescence:

> I was pimply, and my voice was breaking, and I had kind of puppy fat, and I was behaving like a 14-year-old boy. . . . I have a lot of sympathy now for teenage boys because I *struggled* with my brief second male puberty and I had 23 years of life experience leading into it. Plus I'd been socialised as a woman, so I had pretty good communication skills. Twenty-three years of life experience and still I did some dumb shit and couldn't pull my head in—getting really cranky about things and biting people's heads off and stomping around for no good reason. . . . I'm a fairly chilled kind of person but suddenly getting the irrits over tiny things and then having a disproportionate level of pissed-offedness about it and wanting to express it in a really quite physical kind of way, like wanting to slam something, punch things . . . and knowing in my *brain* that I was being an idiot but not being able to control it. I think, if you're the average 13–14-year-old boy who doesn't have all of those other life skills and you don't know what's going on. . . . How any teenage boy makes it through, I think is pretty remarkable. It's not surprising that boys end up in fights.

When a female-to-male (FTM) transsexual person starts taking testosterone, it causes various physical changes: his voice drops, his clitoris enlarges, his breasts shrink, menstruation stops, and hair starts growing in unaccustomed places. For Aram, the fortnightly injections allowed him to grow a beard but also meant asking his (highly amused) girlfriend to wax the unwelcome crop of black hair that appeared on his back. He believes the hormone changed him in less visible ways too, from speeding up his metabolism to inhibiting his emotional responses. He is not the only trans man to tell me the hormone caused his libido to go "monumentally through the roof."

"That kind of thing where all of a sudden you'd be turned on even though you'd been sitting at your desk working," he says, laughing. "I wasn't thinking *anything*, I didn't see *anything*, and all of a sudden I have an issue. And I actually can't concentrate on my work anymore until I go and find something to do about it. Understanding why men are obsessed about sex because now I'm obsessed about sex too and I just am, it's not because. . . . I just *am*. . . . I had a reasonable libido before, but now it's a *lot* more."

His testosterone levels peak about four days after each injection, he says, and he always knows it's happening because of the accompanying increase in sex drive.

Before he became a man, Aram believed gender was mostly a social construct but, having observed the impact of testosterone on himself, he's no longer so sure. "I found myself doing things that were stereotypically male and it genuinely wasn't because I was trying to," he says. Although he sees the core of his personality as having remained fairly constant, some "masculine" qualities have become more pronounced and he has no doubt it's a result of the hormones. He's more restless, impatient, energetic, falls asleep straight after sex and has developed male refrigerator blindness—"If I can't immediately see it, it's too hard to keep looking, it's starting to annoy me and I don't want to look for it any more." More seriously, he says he has lost the ability to cry. The emotional build-up is there but the tears just won't come:

> There's times when it would just be great to cry and just kind of nothing happens. It's pretty awful. You kind of just feel like you need to go bleah and it just doesn't happen. The more emotionally upset I get, the more I end up being *angry*. So I know that I will try really hard now to avoid ever getting very emotionally upset because, once I'm there, I've got an emotion I can't do much with. So I'll be perceived as not engaging and not wanting to talk, but it's actually because I'm trying not to end up in that angry place. Because I can't hit you, and I can't throw things, so I'd rather stay here where things are under control 'cos once I'm over there I'm in trouble. I had to learn to pick when I was starting to get irritable and develop new ways of dealing with emotions because my old ways didn't work anymore.

Is it possible that one small steroid compound could so profoundly affect somebody's personality and behavior? Are men slaves to their hormones, prevented by them from crying (and from finding things in the fridge without female assistance)? I put these questions to Jeffrey Zajac, an endocrinologist who has devoted much of his career to the study of the androgens, or male hormones.

He's skeptical. It's hard to separate any effects hormones might have from the psychological changes that can occur during transition, he says. And there's not much evidence for a link with most of the behaviors we tend to associate with testosterone—not even for aggression, perhaps the one we most take for granted. Transsexual people can't help having expectations about how their new sex is *supposed* to behave and the fact that they are likely to be feeling more comfortable in their bodies, perhaps for the first time in their lives, could contribute to positive changes such as increased energy levels. Although men with abnormally low testosterone do gain increased energy with supplements, there is no reason to suppose a switch from estrogen to testosterone would have the same effect, Zajac says. "I don't think that males in general have more energy than females." The inability to cry he suspects is a social construct, an extension of the belief that boys don't cry. And as for male refrigerator blindness: "It's a nice story. . . . I wouldn't be convinced."

Of all the changes Aram has observed, the one Zajac thinks is most likely to be directly attributable to testosterone is that intrusive sex drive. Although the endocrinologist is not convinced by claims testosterone at lower doses can be used to treat a failing female libido, he thinks it is possible it would have an effect in a genetic female if given at a male dose. One study of transsexual people in transition found the FTM people given testosterone reported increased libido, while the reverse was true for male-to-female people given androgen suppressants and estrogen. Zajac says there's no doubt low testosterone has a negative effect on men's libido:

> In males, if you take their testosterone down to nothing—if they have testicular disease, pituitary disease, they have their testicles removed, or they have treatment for prostate cancer—their libido would go down to nothing. Give them back testosterone, libido goes back up the next day . . . and the wife comes in next time smiling. It's one of the little miracles in medicine.

WEATHERING THE HORMONAL STORM

Testosterone is only one of the hormones constantly coursing through all of our bodies, male or female. Produced by various glands and other organs, these chemical messengers run through the bloodstream from their place of origin to become active in other parts of the body that have the receptors needed to read them. The word hormone comes from the Greek meaning "I arouse" or "I excite," which seems appropriate not just for testosterone: think adrenaline or the so-called stress hormone, cortisol.

The substances we call the sex hormones are a group of closely related steroid compounds derived from cholesterol. They include testosterone and the other androgens, as well as the female hormones estrogen and progesterone. As we saw in chapter 1, the androgens play a crucial role in the physical development of male fetuses and possibly also in brain development, where they are hypothesized to differentiate the male brain from the "default" female option. Androgens also guide the physical changes that happen during male puberty, while the "female" hormones play a similar role in pubescent girls, prompting breast and genital development. In both sexes, the rapidly changing hormone levels contribute to emotional upheaval and the surge of adolescent desire.

I'm using quotation marks because some people question the generally accepted labels, pointing out that not all the functions of these hormones are related to sex and that the "male" hormones are active in female bodies and vice versa. Testosterone and estrogen levels rise in both sexes at puberty, for example, although the balance between the two is different in boys and girls. Pubertal testosterone promotes bone and muscle growth in both sexes and is responsible for the emergence of pubic and underarm hair.

Confusing the picture further is the fact that these closely related hormones have remarkable abilities to turn into each other, even across gender boundaries. For example, the classic female hormone, estrogen, is actually made *from* testosterone. For simplicity's sake, we say the ovaries make estrogen but in fact they first make testosterone and then convert it into the female hormone. This conversion process happens in men too. Whatever testosterone does in male brains, it can only do after it has first been converted to estrogen by an enzyme called aromatase that is present in the brain. So, if the male brain is masculinized by hormonal activity, as most neuroscientists believe, that masculinizing process is carried out by a so-called *female* hormone.

Levels of the different sex hormones vary hugely between people, and also within each of us, in response to environmental factors such as stress, cyclical fluctuations, or normal aging. Male testosterone production, for example, may be at its lowest in late afternoon, while female hormone levels go up and down over the course of the menstrual cycle. Production of the sex hormones declines with age, dramatically for women at menopause, more gradually for men from their thirties on.

Older men can actually have higher estrogen levels than postmenopausal women, but there are clear differences between the adult sexes when it comes to testosterone. The range considered clinically normal for men is around 10 to 30 nanomoles per liter (nmol/L), while for women levels are generally below 2.5 nmol/L. Testosterone levels in the two sexes only overlap in the presence of medical conditions that suppress production in men or boost it in women. By far the most common cause of testosterone deficiency in men in modern Western societies is treatment for prostate cancer, followed by Klinefelter's syndrome (the intersex condition described in chapter 3 that sees men with one or more extra X chromosomes develop small testes that produce lower levels of the hormone). In women, testosterone is produced by the adrenal glands that sit on top of the kidneys and a tumor in these can stimulate testosterone production to near-male levels. Women in this situation can experience a range of masculinizing effects and adrenal tumors in utero are one cause of intersex conditions in genetic females.

Neuroscientist Lesley Rogers sees the hormones as sitting "at the interface of nature and nurture"—they affect our physical and psychological states and those states, in turn, influence the production of hormones in a continuous feedback loop. The stereotype of the testosterone-fuelled warrior is probably inaccurate because stress is one environmental factor that can actually reduce testosterone production in men. In U.S. soldiers during the Vietnam war, for example, testosterone levels were found to be markedly lower just before they embarked on a mission than they were during rest periods. Sexual activity, or even just thinking about sex, has the opposite effect, boosting testosterone production in men. So does winning a tennis game, while losing suppresses production of the hormone.

A number of studies have suggested men's testosterone levels also go down when they become parents, perhaps as a means of encouraging nurturing behaviours. One recent study went further, finding that the more time men spent caring for their children the lower their testosterone went. Direct care of dependent children appeared to actually suppress testosterone production, the researchers wrote.

As well as short-term fluctuations, women also experience regular changes in hormone levels over the course of the menstrual cycle, changes that sometimes seem to be portrayed as *the* force that controls women's lives—a "hormonal windstorm" that makes them emotional, unpredictable, and irrational. This can infuriate women, as any man who has said, "Is it that time of the month?" in the course of an argument has probably discovered. In this view, the hormonal upset of menopause becomes a kind of hurricane, followed by a rather flat and empty calm described by one 1960s medical man in the *Journal of the American Geriatric Society* as "the stigmata of Nature's defeminization." Estrogen supplements could rescue older women from a non-life featuring "eneral stiffness of muscles, a dowager's hump, and a vapid cow-like negative state," Dr. Robert Wilson argued.

Within any individual, shifts in the balance between male and female hormones can lead to physical changes that blur the boundaries between the sexes. Women with higher androgen and lower estrogen levels (because of polycystic ovary syndrome, for example) may develop hard-to-hide facial hair or even a full beard. Molly, a forty-three-year-old former member of the U.S. military, started shaving regularly because of the comments and looks she received:

> I went to the restroom, and this poor little old white lady was coming out of the women's room and giving me the look. She was kind of upset, wondering, trying to say to me that I was in the wrong place, and I felt bad that I was upsetting this old woman. . . . I just kind of thought, "Oh gosh, why am I torturing people like this?" I just didn't like why people were confused, you know, and after a while I just didn't feel like having that kind of attention and confusing people and upsetting them. It wasn't worth the trouble.

And here's Emily, a thirty-two-year-old graduate student, describing the impact of having facial hair on her sense of gender identity:

> It's definitely this sort of crossing over or it's a sort of ambivalence about who I am and the boundary that I've crossed that isn't typical. I don't know how to describe it other than it's sort of a jolt seeing myself with shaving cream [on my face]. . . . [I]t reminds me of my father. . . . [H]aving facial hair is like crossing the boundary between feminine and masculine. It's a perfect example of why our categories shouldn't be so set in our minds of what that is. What's normal or what's freakish? What's masculine? What's feminine? We all have ways that we cross those boundaries, and this is just a major way that we do cross the boundary between masculine and feminine.

Males with higher levels of estrogen can find themselves growing breasts, particularly during the hormonal upheavals of puberty. Although one young man I know joked that he had "lost his feminine side" after having his gynaecomastia—a small lump of female breast tissue—surgically removed, others are less relaxed about the condition. Britain's *The Independent* newspaper in 2009 reported a surge in male breast reductions in that country, some of them no doubt obesity related. One man told the newspaper about the social impact of his man boobs, or "moobs," before he too sought a surgical solution:

> If you're in a group of blokes and they're all macho and there's one of you with moobs, who do you think is going to get picked on? You laugh and joke with them but, deep down, it's mentally wrecking. I have sat at home thinking I wouldn't go out for the rest of my life . . . nobody was going to see my body, no way. I hated everything from the neck down.

Paradoxically, taking male hormones can also lead to unwanted breast development. Because of the body's ability to convert testosterone into estrogen, body-builders and others who take black-market testosterone can be particularly at risk of this kind of feminization. To get rid of unwanted mammary tissue, they sometimes end up taking aromatase inhibitors, breast cancer drugs designed to suppress estrogen production in the breast. Thousands of allied prisoners of war at the end of World War II perhaps faced an even greater challenge to ideas of what constituted a male body. After a long period of stress and malnutrition, some of these men's endocrine (hormonal) systems were so disrupted that a return to normal nutrition saw them start to produce breastmilk. One observer noted five hundred cases of lactation among survivors of a single Japanese POW camp.

THE MYTHOLOGY OF T

Of all the sex hormones, testosterone is the one that seems to have taken on an almost mythological status. As biologist Anne Fausto-Sterling skeptically puts it: "Aggression, violence, crime, riots, war: we owe all these and more to that simple cholesterol-like molecule called testosterone. Or so some would have us think."

Sometimes touted as a "fountain of youth," testosterone is injected by people trying to stave off the aging process or cure a multitude of other ills. Anxious middle-aged men can do quizzes online to tell them if they are going through the "andropause," the (non-existent, according to experts) male equivalent of the female menopause. No prizes for guessing that the motivation behind such websites is to sell hormones to vulnerable men. Some women use testosterone skin patches in a probably misguided attempt to restore an ailing libido, while others apparently inject it for sexual kicks, including its enlarging effect on the clitoris. And the hormone is praised or blamed for a whole range of behaviors and qualities from aggression to the alleged superiority of men in mathematics.

One researcher has come up with a theory that testosterone might actually act as a kind of vaccine against "femaleness" in the developing male. Health sociologist Richard Udry studied women exposed to higher testosterone levels in utero and found they not only engaged in more "cross-gender" behaviors, but were also more resistant to female socialization during childhood than were other girls. In fact, maternal efforts to make them wear dresses and play with dolls actually seemed to push these girls in the other direction. Fetal testosterone might be "immunizing" such girls—and by implication all boys—against feminizing efforts, he concluded:

> Our results indicate that most females are to some degree responsive to variations in gender socialization and so would respond by displaying more masculine or less feminine behaviour. Those highly androgenized prenatally would already have more masculine behavior. But if males being males, are highly immunized against feminine socialization experiences, then attempts at feminizing their socialization would be less effective.

Evidence for most of the behavioral effects of testosterone is actually pretty
sketchy, says Jeffrey Zajac. Although he believes the hormone is likely to
play a structuring role in the brain during early development, particularly in
relation to formation of gender identity and sexual orientation, the picture is
not clear for some of the claimed more far-reaching effects such as cognitive
differences between the sexes. And the evidence for the much-touted link
between testosterone and aggression just isn't there, Zajac says,

> Sure, it's true in cows. If you take testicles off bulls, they're not bulls anymore,
> they're steers. But in humans it's not that clear. . . . The concept that the
> bodybuilders take 10 times as much testosterone and they have these 'roid
> rages, the evidence for that is very weak. Certainly, going from low testoste-
> rone to testosterone replacement, I don't notice an increase in aggression in
> patients I treat. It's not testosterone that makes you aggressive.

It is clear though that the hormone plays a role in early neural development
and function, at least in animals. In some species of birds, the development of
parts of the brain used in courtship songs is dependent on testosterone. Female birds don't show the same neuronal development and they don't sing
the songs. A number of researchers have tried to find similar patterns in
humans, with claims for the effects of fetal hormones ranging from formation
of sexual orientation, to cognitive skills such as spatial orientation, childhood
play preferences, and motivation to pursue a career.

    One of the first hurdles such research faces, however, is that defining
"normal" male and female behaviors in humans is a lot more complex than it
is in songbirds. Various researchers have developed tests designed to provide
objective measures of sex-specific behavior, with questionable results. The
Minnesota Multiphasic Inventory, for example, concluded in 1964 that male
African-American prisoners were more feminine than white males. Some of
the questions used to reveal this hidden female nature included, "Would you
like to be a singer?" and "Do you feel things more intensely than most
people?"

    Psychoanalyst Erik Erikson commented: "That a test . . . singles out as
'feminine' the wish to be a singer and feeling 'more intensely than most
people do' suggests that the choice of test items and the generalizations
drawn from them may say at least as much about the test and the testers as
about the subjects tested." Erikson incidentally was anything but a champion
of androgyny, sighing about the youth of the 1960s: "Sexual identity confusion? Yes, indeed; sometimes when we see them walking down the street it is
impossible for us to tell, without indelicate scrutiny, who is a boy and who is
a girl."

    Tests of gender identity still in use today also raise questions about the
assumptions behind them. The Bem Sex Role Inventory, originally devised
in the 1970s by psychologist Sandra Bem, was one of the measures used in

the Udry study of fetal testosterone and is still sometimes used in clinical settings as one means of evaluating gender identity in people with intersex conditions. I'm not sure which sex should be more offended by the assumptions it makes about our essential natures. Men would be more likely to be classified as feminine if they acknowledged being cheerful, affectionate, loyal, compassionate, tender, sensitive to others' needs, or loving children. Women would be more likely to be considered masculine if they described themselves as self-reliant, athletic, analytical, decisive, competitive, had leadership ability, or defended their own beliefs. Tests like this, with all their assumptions about what constitutes a man or a woman, used to be one of the tools clinicians wielded to decide whether a transsexual person should be allowed treatment or not—too bad for the male-to-female transsexual person who didn't conform to female stereotypes.

Another challenge for researchers attempting to find a connection between hormone exposure and behavior is that a conclusive answer could only be achieved by manipulating fetal hormone levels in humans under controlled conditions—clearly an ethical impossibility. Instead, researchers have to fall back on either animal studies or follow-up of people accidentally exposed to unusual hormone levels in utero. Both have their problems.

When it comes to animals, we can't necessarily assume something that happens in, say, rats will also apply in humans, particularly when it comes to behavior. And defining sex-specific behavior even in animals is not always straightforward either. It's common to read in studies of genetically or hormonally manipulated rats that they demonstrated "male behaviors." Often, what is meant by this is that female or castrated male rats were observed mounting other animals. Having at one point shared my life with several female rabbits who would happily mount anything they could get their front paws on, I find myself wondering if this is really a reliable way of distinguishing male and female behavior in rodents. So I email my old friend Geoff, a professor of the biological sciences who has known a lot of laboratory mice in his time, to ask. He confirms that he has often seen females mount other animals (dogs, cows, mice, rabbits, and guinea pigs to name a few). Scientists usually interpret this as "dominance" rather than sexual behavior, he says, and even by email I can sense a raised eyebrow at the assumptions that might underlie such interpretations by his colleagues.

Even if female rats masculinized by testosterone in utero do mount other animals more frequently than their unmanipulated sisters, this does not have to be a direct effect of the hormone. We are not the only species that socializes our young into gender roles. Mother rats lick sons more often and more vigorously than they do daughters, particularly around the anus and genitals. One study found that mothers with blocked nasal passages, who could not smell the difference between male and female offspring, did not give their boys this extra attention—these males as adults took longer to ejaculate and were capable of less frequent erections. So it is certainly possible that genetically female rats with higher levels of testosterone, and masculinized genitals, might be raised differently from other females.

When it comes to humans, a group that has provided much grist for the research mill is those girls with the intersex condition, congenital adrenal hyperplasia. These girls usually have masculinized genitals at birth because of exposure to high levels of androgens in utero, generally due to a tumor on either their own or their mother's adrenal gland. Various studies have suggested they are more likely to engage in "tomboyish" behavior as children and to have a lesbian sexual orientation as adults, although the findings are not conclusive. Even if these outcomes could be proved, would it necessarily be the testosterone at work? Well, it might play a role but there would certainly be other potential contributing factors. To correct their hormone levels, these girls receive ongoing cortisone treatment and, at least in the past, they routinely underwent genital surgery in early childhood to reduce the size of their clitoris. Either of these interventions could have affected their psychological development. On top of that, the genital ambiguity these girls showed at birth could have had an impact on the way their parents raised them.

The description of a case of adult adrenal hyperplasia in a 1947 medical textbook shows how such conditions tend to be viewed in the context of assumptions about the "natural" behavior of the two sexes: "as the physical changes progressed, [the patient] lost sexual feeling and womanly modesty," the textbook said. However, once the tumor on this woman's adrenal gland was removed, "she became modest and sexually normal, and finally every sign of masculinity, mental and physical, evoked by the tumor vanished." Losing sexual feeling *and* modesty at the same time seems quite an achievement.

More recent claims for behavioral effects of hormones can be just as surprising. One study, for example, suggested moving into work roles that required more aggression and control behaviors had raised testosterone levels in a whole generation of post-feminist women and this might be the cause of higher divorce rates in industrialized nations. From home wrecker to fountain of youth, there are no limits, it seems, to what that small cholesterol-like compound can do.

Chapter Nine

Across the Divide

Standing in Hyde Park in the center of Sydney, beneath century-old fig trees, is a person who cannot be neatly labeled as he or she. Tall and strong-jawed, he looks to me as though he would have been born male so I will use the male pronoun, although it seems inadequate. Naked from the waist up, apart from striped pink arm warmers, he reveals the budding breasts of a pubescent girl beneath the face of a middle-aged man (albeit one who is wearing eye shadow). He has shoulder-length blond curls, a tattooed upper body that, today, is covered in pink body paint, the pot belly of a middle-aged man and white lacy underpants that reveal a more feminine bottom and thighs with a touch of the cellulite that bedevils most women.

It's Mardi Gras time in Sydney, a two-week-long party that some claim is the world's biggest celebration of sexual and gender diversity. Just hours before the festival's famed street parade, the park is thronged with feathers and spangles, with black leather and chains, with naked bottoms and breasts—and a lone optimist bearing a scrawled sign that reads "Jesus is not a myth." There are tourists, too, families in from the suburbs pointing out the most outrageous costumes to their children, and hordes of (very giggly) young women wanting to pose for photographs with the naked men.

"You have a great ass, I mean arse," a plump American tourist says to the almost naked man whose bottom she is about to press her own facial cheek against with a saucy smile for the camera. "You spend a lot of time at the gym, right? Squats and that. I mean, I'm 20 years old and I'm never going to have an ass like that."

"No, honey, you're not," you can almost hear the man thinking, but he grins obligingly, wiggling his bum to give her an extra thrill.

The man in the pink body paint happily lines up for photographs with groups of young women. The whole thing is making me uncomfortable, though it's clearly not having the same effect on him. Perhaps it's those little breast buds, with their hint of puberty, that make me feel as though the gaze of all these fully clothed sightseers is intrusive, even indecent. It is only much later that I wonder about my own assumptions: that he was a pre-op male-to-female transsexual person taking hormones, that this intermediate body was a work in progress, that there was something distasteful about the staring crowds. Perhaps, I think later, what I have seen as an in-between state is actually for this person the end-point. The male physique, the blond curls, the budding breasts, maybe they are all *meant* to coexist and to be exposed to the public gaze. Later again, I find myself wondering if my unease in the park that day was less about the voyeurism of the crowd and more about the fact that I could not easily classify this person's almost naked body as one thing or the other. Why should I have felt the need to protect him from a gaze that did not seem to be bothering him at all?

Our urge to fit people into those male and female boxes can be hard to resist. Sociologist Cecilia Ridgeway writes, "It is striking that people are nearly incapable of interacting with one another when they cannot guess the other's sex."

As part of an attempt to understand how we go about deciding which sex somebody belongs to, psychologists Suzanne Kessler and Wendy McKenna have designed some simple research "games." They created line drawings of naked composite people, mixing and matching male and female characteristics, including genitals, breasts, hip shapes, long or short hair. Then they asked people to identify the sex of these hybrid figures. Male qualities trumped female every time, they found. When genitals were covered, the figures were identified as male 69 percent of the time, despite the actual mix of male and female characteristics across the board being 50-50. Take off their pants and the results were even more striking. Figures with a penis were identified as male 96 percent of the time, but those with a vagina were seen as female only 64 percent of the time. The rule, in Western societies, they concluded was, "*See someone as female only when you cannot see them as male.*" There were no cues that were definitely female, they found, while there were many that were definitely male. "To be male is to 'have' something and to be female is to 'not have' it." Dr. Freud would have been proud.

Kessler and McKenna also devised what they called the Ten Question Gender Game, something a bit like Twenty Questions, in which participants were allowed to ask ten yes/no questions about an imaginary person with the aim of identifying their sex. The only questions they were not allowed to ask were whether the person was male or female. The game was a bit of a trick as the researchers did not actually have a person of either sex in mind and simply answered with a pre-determined series of random yeses and nos.

Participants were asked to keep up a running commentary on which sex they thought the person was after each answer and why. Most players did not ask about genitals—they thought this would have been "cheating" since genitals and gender were clearly the same thing. The two players who asked whether the person had a vagina followed the question with one about a penis, whereas none of the fifteen people who asked about a penis asked a follow-up question about a vagina. Some people who asked the penis question refused to continue the game after that point since they had "the answer."

All of this makes me question my assumption that the man in pink body paint was, in fact, a man. I couldn't see his genitals—if he had a penis, I would guess it was taped back out of sight as the white lacy underpants didn't hide much—but I could see his breasts and feminine clothing. In spite of all the ambiguities he presented, I somehow made a decision to view him as male.

Kessler and McKenna's research casts an interesting light on the fact that female-to-male (FTM) transsexual people often find it easier to "pass"—to convince others they belong to the sex they have transitioned to—than do male-to-female (MTF) people. Until now, I have assumed this simply represents physical differences between the sexes. Trans men can, and most do, grow a beard, a clear marker of maleness. And it is easier for us to accept a slightly built person as a man than it is to see somebody with very large hands and feet, or a masculine jawline, as female. But now I'm wondering if such explanations really cut it. After all, while trans men have beards, trans women have breasts and they also have access to clearer gender markers in dress than their male counterparts. It would seem to make sense for Westerners to assume somebody wearing a skirt and lipstick was female, rather than thinking they were a man in a frock. Yet we don't always do this. If female is the default biological sex, as was suggested in chapter 1, it seems as though male may be the default social one.

"Passing" can be a challenge for both sexes, of course. Going out in public for the first time in a new sex is daunting. And there's always that vexed issue of which toilet you use. At what point during transition do you make the switch? And what if somebody challenges your right to be there?

Karen is somebody who has faced exactly that dilemma. The male-born administrative assistant has been taking female hormones for six months and is still "Matthew" at work, although she is now living as Karen the rest of the time. The impression I get when we meet is of an unremarkable looking middle-aged woman in jeans, white tennis shoes, and a loose black overcoat, but it has taken Karen most of her forty-nine years to find the courage to appear like this in public. Keen to be reassured that she looks "all right" she is still working out the best ways to behave in her new role.

"I've learnt to realise that you actually become more obvious the more you try and hide," she explains. "I mean the first time I walked down to the shops, I think I really made it worse for myself. I'd been to this shop as a guy, and I'm going back to buy some things as Karen, and I'm walking down the street, and some people were walking towards me, and I thought, 'Oh my god, I can't do this,' and I turned around and walked the other way. And I think to myself, 'Oh my god, I've just made a fool of myself, I've made myself *more* obvious by doing that.'"

Using the women's toilets for the first time was a milestone:

> I was in a shopping centre and I *had* to go to the bathroom. I watched and I thought it's quiet now I'll just duck in, sort of really self-conscious, but I thought, well, I can't go into the men's the way I'm dressed. So I popped into the ladies' and I'm sitting there and the next minute I heard these women come in. And one woman says, "Oh, there's only one free." So she popped in and I'm sitting there thinking, oh my god. And then the other one says, "I wonder how long she's going to be. No, I'm still waiting, she hasn't come out yet." It seemed like ages but it was probably no more than a minute. I thought, I've got to do this, I've got to come out. So I opened the door and as I'm coming out she said, "Oh, thank you." And in she went, and it made me realise that she's not worried about me, people just want to get on with their own lives. I know it probably sounds silly but it was a big change. I just felt, no one's going to beat you with a stick.

A few months down the track, Karen delights in stories about occasions when she has successfully passed: the man who opened a door for her, the waiter who said, "Are you girls ready to order?" When she heard a passer-by on the street say, "Was that a man or a woman?" she thought she must be doing something right if they had to guess. Even being abused as a lesbian by passing rednecks when she was giving a female friend a goodbye hug on the street gave her a certain pleasure ("I never thought someone would call me a bloody dyke!"). Perhaps her favorite incident was when she rang to make an appointment to have her legs waxed at an unfamiliar beauty salon. On the phone she had, with trademark diffidence, told them she was transgender and asked if that was OK. When she turned up for the appointment, she was thrilled to be asked, "So, are you going to become a man?"

One thing she has had to learn is not to overdo her attempts to convince others: "Like not getting all dolled up to go down to the shops. Dressing for the occasion, I think that's half the battle. Or make-up . . . I hope it doesn't look too bad today?" She raises an anxious hand to her face but, in fact, her make-up is subtle, just some light foundation and a smear of pale pink lipstick. "I mean going overboard with big eyeshadow," she continues. "I think because you're trying to overcompensate. 'Oh my god, I'd better put more on. I'd better look more feminine.' In reality, what you're doing is pancaking it on and you look worse."

Kessler and McKenna's research suggests transsexual people may indeed find it easier to pass if they don't try too hard to act the part. Players of the Ten Question Game did everything they could to accommodate discordant information within a gender attribution, the researchers found. "All players were able to make sense out of the apparent inconsistencies in the answers, such that players were led to postulate bearded women and men who were transvestites," they wrote. For transsexual people seeking to "pass," the two psychologists suggested first impressions were crucial as "almost nothing could discredit a gender attribution" once it had been made:

> It is not the particular gender which must be sustained, but rather the sense of its "naturalness," the sense that the actor has always been that gender. . . . Gender attributions are so impervious to change that the person will be seen as "crazy" long before she/he is seen as being the other gender.

Our reluctance to let go of a gender attribution once made goes back, perhaps, to that process of learning gender in early childhood when, as we saw in chapter 5, we learn that people's sex does not change just because they put on different clothes or do different things. Transsexual people know only too well how hard it can be to persuade those who have known them for a long time to accept their change of identity. But the research does suggest they might find it easier to establish their gender with people they meet after transition. As long as our first impression of a trans woman was that she was female, she could act as blokey as she liked after that and we would be very reluctant to change our minds.

"A SECRET FEELING . . ."

One patient who sticks in the memory of psychiatrist Louise Newman was a little boy whose parents first brought him to see her when he was five.

"I have a secret feeling," the child said and walked over to whisper in her ear: "I am a girl."

For this boy, the feelings were not new. He had been hiding his penis since he was two or three, saying he didn't like it, and had told his mother he dreamed about being a girl and wanted to be like his younger sister. Starting at primary school had been traumatic—he was afraid of the boys and was teased after telling other children he was a girl.

Newman stresses such behavior does not mean a child will necessarily grow into a transsexual adult, but what we do know is that most transsexual people develop their cross-gender identity early, as we saw in the legal case surrounding "Brodie" that sparked the writing of this book. Children with what clinicians refer to as "gender identity disorder" generally from a very young age reject the label that applies to their biological sex ("I'm not a boy. I'm a girl!"), insist on dressing like a member of the other sex, want to play with children of that sex, and often show distaste for their genitals.

Nobody knows what causes such a radical disjuncture between anatomy and identity, one that has proved utterly resistant to attempts to "cure" it with psychotherapy. The researchers and clinicians I speak to mostly speak in vague terms of a "switch" being turned the wrong way, probably in utero, though some suspect those male hormones are the key. Imaging studies have suggested the brains of MTF transsexual people may be structured in a more "female" than a male way, something that could possibly be due to reduced androgen activity in the developing fetus. Other studies have suggested FTM transsexual people are more likely to have higher androgen levels than most biological females. A group of researchers in Melbourne and Los Angeles have identified one possible genetic contribution—some trans women had genes inhibiting the action of the androgen receptors, meaning their bodies would make less effective use of testosterone.

Whatever the interacting roles of genes, hormones and environment, transsexual people and researchers are united in believing biology plays a big part. In fact, they often describe transsexualism as a kind of "intersex condition of the brain" (though intersex people are not always comfortable with this).

"I'm convinced it's biological," says endocrinologist Jeffrey Zajac. "It's so potent, it's got to be biological. The odds are it's in utero. If it's testosterone that makes you think you're male, then it's that some part of the brain that responds to testosterone isn't responding properly because of some genetic abnormality, that would be my bet."

The transsexual people I speak to in the course of writing this book all say they were aware of their difference from a very young age. Karen would go to bed when she was small, in a nightie surreptitiously taken from one of her sisters, and dream that she would wake up as a girl and "everything would be all right." Norrie May-Welby, as a little boy, fantasized about being Supergirl and never stopped to think that her "bits" didn't correspond with that character, any more than she worried about not coming from Krypton. Aram believed he would one day be an elder of his family's Jehovah's Witness church: "At no point did I go, 'Actually, that doesn't work. Like, you're a girl. You can't grow up to be a male elder with a wife and kids.'" Another man, Craig, remembers being confused when his mother corrected strangers who assumed he was a boy: "If everyone else knows I'm a boy, why do you keep telling them I'm not?" And Peta, a forty-six-year-old beauty therapist and self-described transgender lady, remembers secretly dressing in her mother's clothes:

> I would go into Mum's room and I'd try on her pearl earrings. . . . I just remember *loving* the fashions of the '60s, and Mum had this little pillbox hat made out of feathers and I would put it on, and this coat that she had and I would look in the mirror. I was like seven years of age and I looked in the mirror and I looked like a girl! And I remember thinking, "Oh, my God." It was almost like recognising that that was the real me. But you also instinctively knew that was wrong. So you never talked about it, never did it when anyone else was home.

If childhood was confusing for these children, puberty was something else again. Sexual health physician Darren Russell has observed something he calls the "ugly swan syndrome" at the approach of puberty in genetic boys who believe they are female: "They have this magical belief that they will sprout breasts and long hair and instead they find their voice deepening, and their penis getting bigger, and their body getting hairier."

Adolescents who don't get help at this time can be at serious risk of self-harm, clinicians tell me. For girls who want to be boys, menstruation poses a particular suicide risk as this so fundamentally challenges their sense of who they are. "They routinely cut their wrists at the time of their period," says endocrinologist Garry Warne, who has supported several such children in court when they have sought hormonal treatment to prevent puberty. Although he understands that many people find such an approach confronting, Warne believes the risk of not treating a young person in this situation outweighs the concerns: "You have a child saying I'm going to throw myself under a tram unless you do this for me."

For Karen, puberty was devastating: "I just felt that this is *wrong*. I'm becoming *more* like a boy. I really didn't know who I was. I know what I wanted to be. I just felt so isolated. 'Oh my God, am I the only one that feels like this?' I didn't know where to turn, I just was so upset."

Peta remembers being badly bullied, until she learned to make herself "invisible." Two boys bashed her badly one day after school: "I came home bloodied and bruised and swollen. And Mum said, 'Stay in your room. Don't let your father see you. Don't tell anyone. Keep it to yourself.' And I had to go to school the next day."

THE BODY

Some, though not all, transsexual people will eventually decide to change their bodies so that they better fit their sense of self.

For male-to-female (MTF) transsexual people, this generally means taking female hormones, and possibly an androgen suppressor, before eventually proceeding to surgery. Although the hormones cause some breast growth, they often only produce the small conical breasts of a pubescent girl, so many women choose to have implants.

The most common technique for creating a vagina is known as "penile inversion," essentially a recycling of much of the male equipment to produce a set of female genitals. The penis is dissected and partly removed—blood and nerve connection to a small part of the glans penis is preserved so this can be turned into a sensate clitoris (owners of such organs have told me theirs is capable of orgasm, but studies suggest that is not always the case). Tissue from the outer layers of the penis is used to line the new vagina, which is inserted behind the prostate. Surgeons have to be careful not to include any erectile tissue as this could cause the vagina to constrict, or even bulge outwards, during arousal and the transplanted tissue must also be epilated to prevent hairs from growing inside the vagina. Women who don't have regular penetrative sex may have to continue using a dilator to keep their vagina open. The female urethra and surrounding tissue is constructed from part of the longer male urethra. Labia minora are usually constructed from penile skin and labia majora from the scrotum after the testes have been removed.

For trans men, the surgical options are more limited. Many will have surgery to remove breast tissue, reduce nipple size and recontour the chest, but nobody has yet worked out how to create a fully functional penis. "I would have lower surgery if I thought it was any good," says Aram. "It's something that I continue to struggle with, in terms of not having a body that feels like it properly aligns. I have good days when it's OK and bad days when it really drives me mad, but I'm just not prepared to sacrifice stuff that works for stuff that may not and frankly doesn't look very good and may or may not have feeling."

Men who do decide to brave phalloplasty (penis construction) face long and complex microsurgery. The new penis is made from a roll of skin and other tissue taken from another part of the body, often the forearm, leaving a sizeable scar. The urethra is extended to the tip of this structure using material from the lining of the vagina. The clitoris is kept in place and incorporated into the base of the new penis with the aim of giving some sensation. The resulting organ allows the man to urinate standing up and may, as one medical text puts it, "achieve rigidity" with the help of a prosthesis. Given the uncertain results, it's not hard to see why men might hesitate.

A less ambitious alternative to phalloplasty is a procedure called metoidioplasty that gives the genitals a more male appearance, though without creating a truly functional penis. Surgeons cut ligaments holding the clitoris in place, allowing it to hang further outside the body. Together with the enlargement generally caused by testosterone, this can create an organ that retains sensation and looks like a small penis, perhaps slightly shorter than a thumb. In both phalloplasty and metoidioplasty, a scrotum is constructed from the labia majora, into which implants can be placed to simulate testes.

Although there have been well-publicized cases of trans people regretting their surgery, even in some cases suing the medical services that provided it, research suggests most people are happy with their decision. A large 1991 review found that fewer than 2 percent of transsexual people had persistent regrets about having surgery, and more recent research suggests such regrets have become even less likely as techniques and outcomes have improved.

One trans man described the transformative effect of his mastectomy, despite the pain involved: "I didn't scar as badly as I thought I would and was prepared for. The scars that I do have I wear triumphantly. Like initiation scars worn by some natives as a passage to manhood."

Karen has decided she will definitely have the surgery at some point over the next few years: "I never would have imagined that I *could* do the change physically when I was growing up. That would have been something that couldn't have occurred. I had that thing, and I was born with it, and I was staying with it . . . and then all of a sudden, oh wow, I can do something about it! I'm scared. I'm scared of any surgery but it's something I have to do. I just see that as fulfilling who I am."

It took Peta two decades, during which she went on and off hormones maybe thirteen or fourteen times, to make up her mind to go through with surgery. The hormonal upheaval played havoc with her body and her emotions as she went from growing a beard one month to having milk streaming from her breasts the next. And, each time she stopped the hormones, she rejoiced at the thought that maybe she was finally "cured." Now a happy and rather glamorous woman in her forties, she brushes away tears at the memory of how she felt when she finally had the surgery at age thirty-nine:

> The joy I felt waking up after that operation, it still overwhelms me to this day. For me, it was a rebirth. I've been born twice in this lifetime. I got a second chance at life. I laid in that bed for a week, healing, and in pain, and uncomfortable, but I felt joy.

BEYOND THE BINARY

Transsexualism might seem like the ultimate pulling apart of distinctions between male and female, but in some ways it also reinforces the binary view. If a person has to resort to surgery to make their body fit their sense of who they are, it implies a view that men and women are absolutely, irreconcilably different. As one psychology text puts it, "Children with GID [gender identity disorder] are not androgynous; they are extreme and inflexible in adopting cross-gender but not same gender roles."

I can't help being struck as I talk to transsexual people by the thought that many of them seem to have come from backgrounds where ideas about gender were particularly rigid. Aram's fundamentalist Jehovah's Witness family, for example, believed in principles of male headship of the family and in the church (and the path he has taken has seen him ejected from both). Craig, too, came from a strongly religious background, with parents who were Christian missionaries in the developing world. In Peta's Catholic family, her father was a violent alcoholic with strong views about how his only son should behave. Finding Peta a disappointment on that front, he started sneeringly referring to her as "Mary" while she was still a child.

It's only an anecdotal impression and I'm certainly not suggesting such an environment "causes" transsexualism, but it does make me wonder if something like this might lie behind the much greater prevalence of male-to-female transsexual people, compared with female-to-male. Society's greater acceptance of girls, and women, who adopt behaviors of the other sex might make it easier for females with some level of cross-gender identification to find a place in the world as women. We have traditionally been much more punitive when it comes to males who transgress gender boundaries, perhaps making it harder for some people to see a way of being the person they are while remaining male.

Many transsexual people would reject such ideas because they see their identity as too deeply rooted for it to have been influenced by social factors. And no doubt they are right, at least in relation to their own situation. But the other thing I realize as I talk to people who have been through the experience is that their stories are as varied as those of any other group of humans. Some, far from rejecting their former persona, embrace the qualities of both sexes they observe in themselves. Aram, who describes his current gender as "camp," says his body needed to change but that didn't mean he wanted to change everything about himself:

> Me as a person was me as a person whether I was a boy or a girl. I'd look at these blokey men and I'd go, "Oh my goodness, I don't want to be one of those." I've had to really actively look for men that I can see, "That's kind of me." I found those men more in the gay community. Men that were more

articulate and sensitive, stuff that we usually say is a bit more feminine in a way, masculine men who have emotional language, treat people with respect and don't grunt and that kind of thing.

Aram has wondered if he would have needed to make the physical change if he had grown up in a society that saw gender as something more fluid: "I'd be interested to know if I lived in a different culture at a different time—so exactly me, but somewhere else—I'm sure I would still be kind of male, but would I have had to transition? Like some of the Pacific Islands where there's those biological men who live and are treated and raised as girls, and they never physically transition at all but are just absolutely accepted as women. So there has to be some social stuff in there."

Norrie May-Welby has asked herself the same question. The Sydney artist and activist, who deliberately lives outside binary definitions of sex, says she really likes her androgynous body, produced by a male-to-female sex-change operation but without the additional feminizing influence of hormone therapy. Named "Bruce" at birth, May-Welby had a sex-change operation in her twenties, but stopped taking female hormones soon after. Now, at forty-eight, she has a body that cannot easily be classified as one thing or the other, flat-chested and lean but with "female plumbing."

"If I hadn't had the sex change, would I bother doing it now?" she ponders. "Maybe not, but I'm really happy with the way things turned out for me. It came from being part of this culture that has an obsession about being male or female. I was raised with these ideas. I didn't have alternatives to think about when I went through the operation. I live in a society that is almost intellectually paralyzed by its gender issues. If I was raised in a society that didn't have a hang-up about sex roles, that allowed boys to be feminine and play with dolls, and wasn't homophobic, why would I have bothered to think about surgery? Why would it even be an option my society offered?"

Paradoxically perhaps, May-Welby says she only started to accept her masculine qualities *after* she had the sex change, when she finally gave herself permission to be "a whole human." What did coming to grips with her male nature involve, I ask? "Oh, climbing trees," she says with a laugh. "My thirtieth birthday, I climbed a tree. I've been climbing them ever since. It was a tomboy thing, I guess. A primate thing. Something that girls are told they're not supposed to do."

Transsexual people sometimes say they have been forced to adopt a more rigid identity if they want to convince clinicians they are suitable candidates for surgery. One of the diagnostic criteria used to be that the person was attracted to people of the same biological sex, meaning the operation would make them acceptably heterosexual. May-Welby remembers one doctor who used to stop patients he saw hurrying on the street and admonish them,

"Ladies don't run." Trans man Dean Spade observed others lying and cheating to get through the "medical roadblocks." About his own struggle to convince clinicians to allow him a mastectomy, he wrote:

> In order to be deemed real I need to want to pass as male all the time, and not feel ambivalent about this. I need to be willing to make the commitment to "full-time" maleness, or they can't be sure that I won't regret my surgery. The fact that I don't want to change my first name, that I haven't sought out the use of the pronoun "he," that I don't think that "lesbian" is the wrong word for me . . . is my undoing in their eyes.

Convincing health professionals is only part of the battle. When people transition to a new sex, they also need to get legal authorities to accept their new identity. A bearded man trying to travel on a female passport would probably not have a great time on his overseas trip. Changing legal status can mean jumping through all sorts of hoops. As well as providing medical evidence to show that they have made the required physical changes, in some jurisdictions transsexual people may be required to divorce a partner they married before they transitioned, even if the relationship remains a strong and committed one.

Aram tells me of his desire to challenge such laws. A lesbian before he made the transition to a male sexual identity, he is still in a relationship with the woman he was with before he started taking male hormones, had chest surgery to remove his breasts and grew a beard. Although he has managed to have his passport changed, getting a male birth certificate—required for him to marry a female—is a much bigger challenge. So central is the presence or absence of a penis to our understanding of gender that it tends to be easier for trans women to satisfy the legal requirements. When a biological male has the organ surgically removed, and a vagina constructed, authorities may gulp but they accept that the resulting body belongs to a woman. The more limited surgical options make it harder for those who go in the other direction.

"It's ridiculous," Aram says. "You can't neatly legally define the concept of a man or woman, so then having a law which says marriage is between a man and a woman is kind of stupid. If my girlfriend and I just put in papers today asking to get married we'd be refused because they ask for your birth certificate. They'd see two female birth certificates so they'd say, 'No way.' [But] I reckon if . . . I found a guy and the man and I put in papers they'd go, 'Oh yeah, you can get married,' then we'd rock up at the registry office and they'd go, 'Waaait a minute, what's going on here?' . . . We'd probably end up in court and I don't know which way they'd rule. . . . There's a part of me that would really like to do that as a stunt, apply to marry my girlfriend, get refused and then go round with some boy and apply to marry him just to point out how idiotic it all is."

Norrie May-Welby has perhaps posed an even greater challenge to authorities with her ongoing fight to be legally recognized as not belonging to either gender. To support her case, May-Welby, who lightheartedly describes herself as "a eunuch, biologically neuter," has put forward evidence from several doctors attesting she cannot be classified as one thing or the other. (She has, however, given me permission to use female pronouns when describing her, although she herself would opt for the newly coined gender-neutral terms "zie" for he/she and "hir" for his/her.)

Gender theorist Susan Stryker, herself a trans woman, believes such complexities and ambiguities have helped to create a social "imperative of counting past two," destabilizing traditional definitions of gender and sexual orientation.

I've had to attempt this mathematical feat many times in the course of researching this book, perhaps most radically as a result of my meetings with transsexual people. Their stories have been thought-provoking, moving, occasionally confronting, but that hasn't been the only impact. Waiting to meet these strangers in parks or on city streets has, for me, disrupted the normally unquestioned process of assigning a gender to everybody we encounter. Sitting on a bench waiting to meet a trans man for the first time, I have found myself looking at every passing male, thinking, "Could you have been a woman once?" It's been a disconcerting experience at times, but one that has also helped me to start learning to think in numbers bigger than two.

Afterword

Early in 2009, two young Swedish parents found themselves at the center of a storm of cyber abuse. What had these two twenty-four-year-olds done to deserve being called everything from "laughable and moronic" to "sick fucks"?

They had talked to a newspaper journalist about their decision to raise their child, "Pop," without disclosing his or her sex. When people asked whether the two-and-half-year-old was a boy or a girl, the parents simply said: "We have chosen not to reveal our child's sex."

"We want Pop to grow up more freely and avoid being forced into a specific gender mould from the outset," Pop's mother told Swedish newspaper *Svenska Dagbladet*. "It is not an experiment. I think it is much worse to bring a person into this world with a blue or pink stamp on their forehead."

Whatever you think about this project, the hysterical responses it engendered in some quarters seem a little out of proportion. The parents, known only by the pseudonyms Jonas and Nora, said they were not seeking to deny the child's sex and that it would be up to Pop to decide what and when to disclose. In the meantime, they wished to avoid having others' preconceptions about boys and girls imposed on the child, based on their belief that gender was a social construct.

Personally, I think it sounds like a pretty self-indulgent project that poses some risk of psychological harm to the child, but Nora and Jonas wouldn't be the only parents ever to have done *that*. My guess is Pop will fairly swiftly take matters into his or her own hands and put an end to the whole thing (and probably already has given that by the time this book is published he/she will be approaching school age).

One thing the reaction to Pop's story does highlight is how important sex and gender are to us as ways of classifying people and how uncomfortable we feel when those categories are taken away from us. For all the increased freedom of our Western societies, the greater flexibility about both male and female roles at and outside work, we still seek those reference points of male and female when we think about or interact with other people. And almost all of us use, and *want* to use, those terms to describe ourselves. We learn them early, integrate them into our identities, charge them with extra energy as we become sexual beings, defining ourselves by them even when we resist them. Few of us would actually want to make Norrie May-Welby's choice to live outside the gender binary, although many of us might welcome some blurring around the edges.

Much of this book has been about bodies, about that constant, two-way interaction between biology and environment that helps construct who we are as human beings—the hormones that influence our behavior and are, in turn, influenced by it. Our creative, ever-changing brains that seem, in ways we still don't really understand, to house the very essence of us. Men and women, boys and girls, and those who are somewhere in between, we are all a work in progress, subject to the transformative power of the world around us, and transforming it in our turn.

We have seen so much change over the last half century or so: the shifts in gender roles brought on by the women's movement, by gay liberation, by new technologies such as the Pill, to name a few. In some ways, we have become more androgynous, embracing a wider range of possible behaviors for both sexes, while in others we have proved resistant to change. Faced with the unsettling fluidity of much of modern life, some of us have retreated, seeking comfort in old certainties about the essential natures of men and women. The pace of change seems unlikely to slow any time soon and it's anyone's guess what the next fifty years will bring. Will a conservative backlash see women return to the domestic sphere and men give free rein to their supposed inner cave man? Or will we all become less fixed in our genders as we spend more of our lives in the disembodied world of cyberspace where we can each perform as many identities as we like? Even that most basic biological definition of male and female, as carriers of sperm and eggs, could be undermined as new medical technologies raise the possibility of two men or two women being able to combine their genetic material in the laboratory to produce a child.

Whatever changes might lie ahead, I'm pretty sure sex and gender will always be with us. Why? Because deep down we *like* them. At least, that is the case for those of us fortunate enough to live in relatively liberal societies where the shape of our bodies, and the things we choose to do with them in the company of other consenting adults, does not overwhelmingly determine the way we are allowed to live our lives. We might want to play with our gender, to be free to transgress it at will, but most of us like our gendered bodies with the various sexual and other meanings we attribute to them.

Call me Utopian, but I'd like to see a world where each of us could grow to be the person we wanted to be, without the constraint of stereotypes, sex-based or otherwise. Not a world without men and women, but one where little boys and girls could play together (if they chose), where fathers could take time off to care for children without being discriminated against at work, where men could play football *and* knit on the bus, where women could drive trucks *and* wear high heels (though perhaps not at the same time). And where those people who didn't fit neatly into the binary could find a happy and accepted place.

The online polemicists who predicted Pop would inevitably be driven to suicide in teenage years by the parental meddling with his or her gender identity perhaps need to be more aware that rigid enforcement of the gender binary can also have devastating effects. Several of the transsexual people I met spoke of a lost and lonely adolescence when they felt compelled to attempt suicide because they were unable to fit into the box prescribed for them. Rigid applications of any ideology do not tend to serve children well, something Pop's parents would also do well to keep in mind.

I'm going to leave the final words to a self-identified trans person who commented on the Pop case in an online forum. You may not agree with everything this person says, but it's worth thinking about the kinds of worlds we humans might be capable of creating:

> Although I think the Utopian ideal of a genderless society is perhaps interest-
> ing, I don't think it sounds like a society I'd like to live in. I like gender, I just
> don't like the amount of meaning we attach to it. What if gender carried no
> more meaning than color. What if I wore masculinity today in the same way I
> wore the color green. Gender is a wonderful, amazing, colorful world and
> worth exploring and exploding—much too interesting to get rid of altogether.
> One day perhaps we'll be able to let children choose their gender. . . . Will Pop
> experience some awkward situations? Of course. We all do as children. I only
> hope that if Pop decides that Pop is a totally gender conforming girl or boy that
> Pop's parents will be OK. Sometimes parents get to struggle and push boun-
> daries and sometimes parents have to settle for the fact that their children are
> decidedly and painfully normal and love them in spite of it.

Glossary

5-alpha reductase deficiency An intersex condition in which a chromosomal male is unable to synthesize the testosterone derivative dihydrotestosterone, the hormone responsible for guiding male development in utero, although he is able to make and use testosterone itself like any other male. People with this condition often look female at birth but become much more masculine at puberty because the physical changes that occur then depend on testosterone directly.

androgen insensitivity syndrome (AIS) An intersex condition that sees an embryo with male chromosomes (one X and one Y), testes and male levels of testosterone follow a female developmental path because the receptors that allow the body to use male hormones are not functioning properly.

androgens The so-called male hormones, principally testosterone and its derivatives such as dihydrotestosterone.

anti-Müllerian hormone (AMH) A hormone produced by the Sertoli cells in the testis of the developing male embryo that prevents the female Müllerian ducts from developing.

bipotentiality The ability of various structures within the human embryo to take two different developmental paths, one male, one female (the early phallus's ability to develop into either a penis or a clitoris, for example).

brain plasticity The ability of the brain to rewire itself in response to new learning or experiences.

chimaera An individual created by merging of genetic material from more than one fertilized egg.

chromosomes Structures in the nucleus of cells that group genes together in matching pairs (one copy of each gene from each parent). Cells normally contain 46 chromosomes, apart from the germ cells (the eggs and sperm), which contain 23 each. Two of the 46 chromosomes are sex-determining—males typically have one X and one Y chromosome, while females have two Xs.

congenital adrenal hyperplasia An intersex condition resulting from a baby girl's exposure to high levels of male hormones in utero.

dihydrotestosterone A derivative of testosterone that guides male development in utero.

disorders of sexual development (DSDs) An umbrella term used by clinicians to describe intersex conditions.

endocrine system The organs that produce hormones and the hormones themselves.

gender identity disorder (GID) A clinical term used to describe people whose gender identity does not match their biological sex. (Sometimes called gender dysphoria or *transsexualism*.)

genital ridge The area in the developing embryo that has the potential to become either a testis or an ovary.

genome or **genotype** The total of all the genes in an individual.

germ cell The male sperm or female egg.

gonad The male testis or female ovary.

granulosa cells Cells in the ovary that form the ovarian follicles, protecting and nourishing the developing eggs.

hermaphroditism A term describing people whose sex is chromosomally or anatomically ambiguous. Largely replaced by the term *intersex*, and now considered offensive by many intersex people, it is still occasionally used in clinical literature to describe people who have both testicular and ovarian tissue.

hormones Chemical substances produced in one organ of the body that travel through the bloodstream to become active in a different body part that has receptors to read that particular hormone. The so-called sex hormones are a group of steroid compounds that includes the male hormones (mainly testosterone and its derivatives) and the female hormones (estrogen and progesterone).

hypospadias A condition that sees boys born with the urethral opening on the underside of their penis rather than at the tip, often considered an intersex condition at least in its more severe forms.

intersex A range of medical conditions in which individuals are born with some degree of anatomical or chromosomal sex ambiguity.

Klinefelter's syndrome An intersex condition in which males have one or more extra X chromosomes.

Leydig cells Cells in the testis that produce the male hormone, testosterone.

meiosis The process that sees the primordial germ cell split in two to create two separate sperm (in the male) or eggs (in the female), each carrying half the normal number of chromosomes.

Müllerian ducts The primitive structures that become the Fallopian tubes, uterus, and upper part of the vagina if a developing embryo goes down the female path.

ovary The female gonad, which produces eggs and the hormone estrogen.

ovotestis An ambiguous gonad containing both ovarian and testicular tissue that is found in some intersex conditions.

oxytocin The so-called "feel-good hormone," released, for example, during sex and in parents caring for their small children. It facilitates interpersonal bonding and possibly brain plasticity.

parthenogenesis A process through which some female animals can produce offspring from their own genetic material (effectively, clones) without need for a sexual partner.

primordial germ cell A cell that has the ability to divide into either two sperm or two eggs, depending on whether it finds itself inside a testis or an ovary.

pseudohermaphroditism A term considered offensive by some intersex people but used in scientific literature to describe intersex conditions where the person concerned has only ovaries or testes, rather than a combination of both.

Sertoli cells Cells in the testis that protect and nourish developing sperm as well as inhibiting female development in surrounding cells.

sexual dimorphism The physical differences between the two sexes in a given species.

***Sry/SRY* gene** The so-called male gene or "sex-determining region Y," the gene on the Y chromosome that initiates the process of male development. *Sry* is the mouse gene; *SRY* is the human gene.

testis The male gonad, which produces sperm and the hormone testosterone.

trait In genetics, the effect a gene has when it is expressed, such as blue eyes, for example.

transsexualism A term used to describe people whose gender identity does not match their biological sex.

Turner's syndrome An intersex condition in which women have only one X chromosome.

Wolffian ducts The primitive ducts that can become the sperm-conducting ducts if a developing embryo follows the male pathway.

References

Full details of references cited here can be found in the Bibliography.

PREFACE

There are numerous clips of Semenya's race and interviews with the media on YouTube, and Ariel Levy's article in *The New Yorker* offers an excellent discussion of the case. Jonathon Reeser has written a review of the history of gender verification in sport. Information about female athletes is from chapter 13 of the *IAAF Medical Manual*.

INTRODUCTION

When it comes to feminist theory, Judith Butler has, for example, said the distinction between sex and gender "turns out to be no distinction at all"—if sex itself is a gendered category, it makes no sense to define gender as the cultural expression of sex (p. 10). She also makes the thought-provoking suggestion that gender is better conceived of as something we perform or "do" than as something we "are" (p. 34). It is interesting to wonder how our identities might shift if we said, "I do male," rather than, "I am a man." Tannaz Eshagian's 2008 documentary *Transsexual in Iran* sensitively portrays the dilemmas faced by gay and trans people in that country.

The judgment in the Brodie case is Family Court document no. FamCA 334.

1 CONCEIVING GIRLS AND BOYS

The information about diverse methods of reproduction in animals is from Catton and Gray, pp. 103–10 and 113–14.

Geddes is quoted on p. 184 of Fausto-Sterling's *Myths of Gender*. The description of the process of conception is drawn from Richard Jones, pp. 169–80, and Hunter, pp. 93–95. The creation of sperm and eggs from the primordial germ cells is described by Hunter on pp. 75–76. Early theories of conception and the history of the discovery of the sperm and the egg are described in chapter 1 of Hunter. The preformationist view is outlined by Coen on pp. 2–3.

The research into environmental effects on human sex ratios is summarized in Steve Jones, pp. 45–47. Some studies have suggested older parents have more girls, while mixed-race couples have more boys. It has also been suggested that parents who smoke more than twenty cigarettes a day are less likely to produce sons, with the effect stronger in fathers than in mothers, perhaps because the fragile Y chromosome is more vulnerable to the toxins in cigarettes.

The discovery of the Y chromosome's role in determining sex is described on pp. 13 and 23 of Hunter, while the genetic contribution to sex determination is covered more broadly in the first two chapters of that book. The role of the female in determining sex in birds is outlined by Drews on p. 325. Graves's discussion of the smart and sexy X chromosome is in her 2006 paper, while her appraisal of the Y chromosome is in her 2000 paper.

The role of testosterone in structuring the male brain in animals is described in many scientific texts, including Drews, pp. 325–43. The hormone's role in the human brain is discussed in Ruble and Martin, pp. 965–69. The description of embryonic sex differentiation is drawn from Richard Jones, pp. 117–35; Hunter, pp. 79–96, 107–15; Drews, pp. 325–43; and Larsen, pp. 173–205. The quote about the greater research focus on male development is on p. 58 of Hunter.

2 THE EVOLVING MAN AND WOMAN

James Holland Jones's quote is from his *Monkey's Uncle* blog posting of 23 December 2008. The aims of evolutionary psychology are outlined by Bjorklund and Pellegrini, in a paper that seeks to use the techniques of the evolutionary psychologist to provide insights into child development. A critique of evolutionary psychology's claims—in this case, in relation to evolutionary explanations for detection of cheating, jealousy, and parental love—can be found in Buller's paper. Arguments on both sides are included in the ensuing debate in the letters pages of the same journal, *TRENDS in Cognitive Sciences*; 9:506–7. The description of chimpanzees exchanging meat for sex is in Ridley's *The Origins of Virtue*, pp. 89–91, among others. The way learned behaviors can be passed on from one generation to the next is discussed in Fausto-Sterling's *Myths of Gender*, pp. 199–200.

The descriptions of primate sexuality are from Stanford's paper and the many responses published with it, including that by Ingmanson, whose quote about the bonobos is on p. 409. De Waal is quoted on pp. 407 and 399 of Stanford. The quote from Stanford about our imposition of human sex stereotypes onto the chimps and bonobos is on p. 407. Additional information on primate sexuality is from Dawkins's *The Ancestor's Tale*, pp. 109–16, Steve Jones, pp. 209–15 and Matt Ridley's *Nature via Nurture*, pp. 18–21. The study of gorilla paternity is by Nsubuga et al. The polyandrous birds are described in Fausto-Sterling's *Myths of Gender*, p. 185. Elephant seals and sexual dimorphism are discussed in Dawkins's *The Ancestor's Tale*, p. 210ff. Data suggesting women rate wealth more highly than men do when looking for a mate are summarized in Ridley's *Nature via Nurture*, pp. 53–55. Hitsch et al's study of online dating provides more recent evidence of this and other mate preferences. Evidence of infidelity in monogamous blackbirds has been reported by Garamszegi and Møller and in gibbons by Reichard.

Trut's description of the silver fox experiment was published in *American Scientist* in 1999. Dawkins's quote about the evolution of human tameness is on pp. 31–32 of *The Ancestor's Tale* and his discussion of lactose tolerance is on p. 33. Some research into recent human evolution is reported on by Voight et al. Dawkins discusses sexual selection and the peacock's tail on p. 270ff of *The Ancestor's Tale*. Fausto-Sterling's discussion of species that evolve to fit a narrow ecological niche and the quote about the condor is on p. 170 of *Myths of Gender*.

3 HERMES AND APHRODITE

The quote from Borges is on p. 103 of his essay collection. Foucault's response to it is on p. xv of his book, *The Order of Things*.

Vilain's estimate for the incidence of atypical genitalia at birth is on p. 44. European Association of Urology guidelines suggest the increase in hypospadias may be due to pesticides. In Australia, a West Australian study found 2.8 baby boys in a thousand had hypospadias in 1980, rising to 4.3 per thousand by 2000. The increase was even greater at the more serious end of the spectrum, with moderate to severe cases almost doubling over the period. In an interview with *Australian Doctor*'s Rebecca Jenkins, one of the authors of the study suggested exposure to chemicals such as pesticides might be behind the rise. Klinefelter's syndrome is described on pp. 224–26 of Hunter, while Turner's syndrome is on pp. 220–22. The case of the man with two copies of the *SRY* gene was described by Eric Vilain on p. 53. Chimaeras are described on pp. 245–56 of Hunter. The description of 5-alpha reductase deficiency and its manifestation in different cultures is drawn from Preves, pp. 29 and 40–42.

The extract from the *British Medical Journal* is quoted by Dreger on pp. 59–60 and the Pozzi quote is on p. 70. Drake's advice to pregnant women is on pp. 105–7. Dreger outlines her view of the "age of gonads" on p. 11 and the debate over rectal examinations on p. 92. The two medical texts from the 1990s advocating rearing a child as a female in the absence of an adequate penis are quoted in Diamond and Sigmundson, p. 57. Chase's account of her experiences is on pp. 300–314.

4 THE SEXED BRAIN

I am indebted to Professor Lesley Rogers for drawing my attention to the work of Gustave LeBon. Those who read French can digest the whole paper in the Bibliothèque Nationale de France's wonderful online archive at gallica.bnf.fr. The summary of Broca's career is from Winston, pp. 35–37. The Musée Dupuytren can be visited by appointment.

The relationship between body and brain size in the two sexes is outlined in Rogers's *Sexing the Brain*, p. 7. The research into structural differences between male and female brains is summarized by Cahill in his 2006 review. Winston makes his suggestion that the structure of male brains inhibits expression of feelings on pp. 68–69. Fausto-Sterling's discussion of the corpus callosum research is on pp. 115–45 of her *Sexing the Body* and the quote about old and new approaches to studying the brain is on p. 27. The findings of fMRI and PET studies of the brain are summarized by Cahill. The study of the two sexes' response to cartoons was conducted by Azim et al. Potential clinical applications of a better understanding of sex differences in the brain are discussed by Azim et al, Hoeft et al, and Cahill. The MRI study of male and female intelligence is by Haier et al. Deary et al. are the authors of the review of the neuroscience of intelligence quoted in the final paragraphs of this section.

Baron-Cohen quotes Asperger on p. 149 of his 2003 book, while the quote describing his own conclusions is on p. 1. His discussion of possible evolutionary explanations for the differences he identifies is on pp. 117–31, including the quote about women as poor systemizers on p. 130. His students' research into the attention of newborns is on pp. 55–56. The summary of research on women's supposed greater linguistic ability is also taken from pp. 57–59 of this book. The male/female brain tests are also in his book. The graphs allowing the plotting of individual scores and giving distribution figures for the various brain types are in Baron-Cohen's 2005 paper. Rogers outlines her views on the biological determinism she sees in much scientific research into sex differences throughout her book, *Sexing the Brain*: see pp. 2–3, for example. The quotes here are from her 2003 review of Baron-Cohen's book.

Training different parts of the brain to take over functions once performed in regions damaged by stroke is an exciting area of neurological research: Huxlin et al. report, for example, on successful attempts to train "cortically blind" people to use different parts of their brain to process visual images after damage to the visual cortex. Freeman's argument and the research on brain plasticity more generally is outlined by Doidge; see, for example, p. 118ff. Rogers describes the research suggesting mothers talk more to baby girls than boys on p. 26 of her book, while the quote from her is on p. 25. The longitudinal study of scholastic aptitude was by Feingold.

5 LEARNING GENDER

The account of the John/Joan case, including all the quotes from Reimer himself and the quote from Money about the progress of the case, is drawn from Diamond and Sigmundson's article revealing its outcome. Supplementary material and the account of the difficulties encountered by other family members comes from an article written after Reimer's suicide by his biographer, John Colapinto. Further analysis is provided by Fausto-Sterling in her *Sexing the Body*, pp. 66–71, including the 1972 quote from Money on p. 67.

The summary of research into children's understanding and application of gender stereotypes is drawn from Ruble and Martin, pp. 945–53 and 963–64, including the quote about stereotypes being held rigidly until about age eight, p. 947, and the quote about boys holding more tightly to stereotypes, p. 948. Additional information on gender stereotypes is from Leaper and Friedman, p. 565ff. The exchange between the preschool aide and the boy with the necklace was recorded by West and Zimmerman, p. 209.

The research suggesting we treat baby boys and girls differently is discussed in Ruble and Martin, p. 983 and in Brody, p. 28. The stages in children's understanding and development of gender identity are described in Ruble and Martin, pp. 957–58, 963–65, and 972–96. The same authors discuss childhood gender identity disorder on pp. 952–53 and 963–64. Brody is one of several authors to have suggested little boys need to reject femininity because of the preponderance of female caregivers surrounding them, and the quote is from p. 32 of her paper. Boys' reluctance to follow a female role model is discussed in Ruble and Martin, pp. 972–76. Brody's quote about boys' need to conform to masculine rules is on pp. 26–27, as is her discussion of what makes girls popular. Stoller is quoted in Gilmore, p. 172.

The quote about sex segregation is on p. 994 of Ruble and Martin and the punitive approach to boys who cross gender boundaries is described on pp. 954–58 and 963. The differences in emotional expression between adolescent boys and girls are described on p. 960. Hyde's paper on the gender similarities hypothesis was published in *American Psychologist* in 2005. The studies of aggression are discussed in Ruble and Martin, pp. 959–60. The quote about boys and girls playing together outside school is on p. 189 of Thorne, while the longer quote is on p. 192. His argument that children create culture as well as being formed by it is on p. 196. The quote from Reay is on p. 308 of her paper.

6 THE THIRD AND MANY GENDERS

Donald Brown's list of human universals is included in an appendix to Pinker, pp. 435–39. Oyeronke Oyewumi's work is described in Fausto-Sterling's *Sexing the Body*, pp. 19–20. Evidence that women hunt in various cultures is cited in Brettel and Sargent, p. 202. Eleanor Maccoby points out that women are the load carriers in many cultures on p. 2 of *The Two Sexes*. Lamphere's quote about the public-private dichotomy is on p. 72 of her paper, while the description of Iroquois women's work is on p. 70. The quote from Margaret Mead's book *Male and Female* is in Lamphere, p. 68. The information about women from the Plains tribes is from Walter Williams's essay on "Amazons" in the Americas, and the reference to a woman joining a war party is on p. 185; the Griffins' account of the Agta people is on pp. 206–15.

The description of Masai manhood rituals is in Gilmore, p. 165 and the quote about the nature of manhood is on p. 167. The quote about boys' need to separate from their mother is on p. 172.

An article about the Thai school's toilets appeared on *BBC News*, written by Jonathan Head. Peter Jackson discusses the Western interpretation of Thai gender cultures in his 1999 book, and the quote is on pp. 226–27. Stryker's quote is on p. 14 of the book she coedited with Stephen Whittle. Information about the hijras comes from Herdt, pp. 145–47, and from Nanda's two essays. The quote from Nanda is on p. 550 of her contribution to the reader edited by Abelove et al. The Gandavo quote is from Williams's essay, p. 179. The discussion of two-spirit people, including the information about Mohave males, is from Herdt, p. 93. The information about Mohave females and women in northern tribes is from Williams, pp. 180–83. The quote from Harry Benjamin is on p. 47. Ruble and Martin discuss studies suggesting gay people have more cross-gender interests in childhood on p. 962.

7 SEXING SEXUALITY

The quotes from Fulgence Mayer's booklet, *Safeguards of Chastity,* can be found on pp. 59, 67 and 76. The quote from Kramer and Sprenger's *Malleus Maleficarum* is on p. 47. William Acton is quoted on p. 243 of Roy Baumeister's paper. Janet Shibley Hyde's discussion of sex differences in sexuality is on p. 586 of her paper. The recent review of psychological research is by Baumeister et al. and the quote is to be found on p. 263. The research on differences between gay male and lesbian behavior is discussed on p. 247 of the same paper, while data showing men report more sexual partners than women are presented on p. 250. The difference in the two sexes' claims about the age of loss of virginity are discussed in Alexander and Fisher. The 2007 study of American college students is by England et al. The lie-detector study is by Alexander and Fisher. The global study of sexual behaviors and attitudes is by Schmitt.

Masters and Johnson are quoted in Komisaruk et al's book on the science of orgasm, p. 1, and the study of students' accounts of orgasm is described on pp. 1–7 of the same book. Stopes's quote about male ejaculatory restraint is on pp. 163–64 of her book, *Married Love.* The Dutch research into the orgasmic brain is reported in Georgiadis et al. and Holstege et al. The quote from Holstege is from the *Times* article by Henderson. The physiology of orgasm and the estimated prevalence of female orgasmic difficulty is from Richard Jones et al, pp. 368–75 and 388. Berger and Kroger are quoted by Morgan on p. 81 of her book. Evolutionary explanations for the female orgasm are discussed in Komisaruk et al, pp. 8–15.

The research on pheromones is summarized in Richard Jones, p. 382. The first study of feminized faces is presented in Perrett et al. The follow-up is by Penton-Voak et al. The cross-cultural research suggesting mate preferences change as societies become more egalitarian is reported by Johannesen-Schmidt and Eagly. The study of online dating is by Hitsch et al, and the discussion of male and female mate preferences is on pp. 21–26. The story about Kinsey inserting a swizzle stick into his urethra is recounted in Roach, p. 33. Research on early development of sexual orientation is summarized in Ruble and Martin, pp. 961–62. The study of arousal from male and female sexual stimuli is by Chivers et al, while research into women's sexual plasticity is summarized in Peplau et al.

8 TESTOSTERONE AND FRIENDS

The study of libido in FTM and MTF transsexual people is described in Baumeister et al, p. 266.

Anne Fausto-Sterling, for example, argues the so-called sex hormones should be reclassified as growth hormones to emphasize their role in tissue growth in both sexes. These hormones should not be seen as belonging to one sex or the other, she argues in *Sexing the Body*, pp. 146–94. The information on environmental factors that influence testosterone levels comes from Rogers, *Sexing the Brain*, pp. 75–77. The study of new fathers' testosterone levels is by Gettler et al. The term "hormonal windstorm" is used by Fausto-Sterling in *Myths of Gender*, p. 121. She quotes Wilson's description of the postmenopausal woman in *Sexing the Body*, p. 146. Molly and Emily are two of the women interviewed for Debra Beechy's master's thesis and the quotes can be found on pp. 83–84. The article about moobs appeared without a byline in *The Independent* on 7 March 2009. The information about allied prisoners of war lactating after World War II comes from Jared Diamond's article in *Discover*.

The Fausto-Sterling quote about testosterone is in *Myths of Gender*, p. 126. Some doctors believe women with low libido may benefit from testosterone supplements, although the practice is controversial and the evidence is at best equivocal. Udry's paper makes the suggestion that testosterone might "immunize" men against female socialization on pp. 452–53. The research into testosterone and the neurodevelopment of male songbirds is cited in Fausto-Sterling, *Myths of Gender*, p. 133. The Minnesota Multiphasic Inventory is discussed on pp. 305–7 of Erikson and his quote about androgynous youth is on p. 26. Many studies refer to mounting as an indication of male behavior in rodents. Some of these, along with the description of rat mothers' anogenital licking of their sons, are described in Fausto-Sterling's *Sexing the Body*, pp. 227–30. Studies of girls with congenital adrenal hyperplasia are described in *Sexing the Body* on pp. 73–75 and in *Myths of Gender*, pp. 134–38. The 1947 medical textbook is by Garrod and Thursfield and the case is described on p. 414. The study suggesting women's move into the workforce could have raised their testosterone levels and with them the divorce rate is described in Udry, pp. 444–45.

9 ACROSS THE DIVIDE

Ridgeway is quoted on p. 10 of Wharton. Kessler and McKenna describe their research into gender attribution on pp. 165–82, with the quote about sustaining "naturalness" on p. 177.

The study of the possible genetic contribution to transsexualism was reported by Hare and colleagues. The information on sex-change surgery is from Bowman and Goldberg, pp. 5–26. The research on satisfaction with the surgery is summarized on p. 4 of the same document. The quote from the trans man about his mastectomy is on p. 51 of the report by Couch and colleagues.

The quote from the psychology text about children with gender identity disorder is on p. 950 of Ruble and Martin. Spade described his experience on pp. 315–32 and the quote is on p. 322. Stryker's comments are on p. 8 of the book she coedited with Stephen Whittle.

AFTERWORD

An account of the Pop case in English is given by Parafianowicz. The original Swedish article is by Sjöström. Anna McCredie assisted with translation of the quotes.

Bibliography

Alexander, Michele, and Fisher, Terri. "Truth and Consequences: Using the Bogus Pipeline to Examine Sex Differences in Self-Reported Sexuality," *The Journal of Sex Research* 40 (2003): 27–35.

Azim, Eiman et al. "Sex Differences in Brain Activation Elicited by Humor," *Proceedings of the National Academy of Sciences* 102 (2005): 16, 496–501.

Baron-Cohen, Simon. *The Essential Difference: The Truth about the Male & Female Brain.* New York: Basic Books, 2003.

Baron-Cohen, Simon et al. "Sex Differences in the Brain: Implications for Explaining Autism," *Science* 310 (2005): 819–23.

Batty, David. "Mistaken Identity," *The Guardian*, 31 July 2004.

Baumeister, Roy et al. "Is There a Gender Difference in Strength of Sex Drive? Theoretical Views, Conceptual Distinctions, and a Review of Relevant Evidence," *Personality and Social Psychology Review* 5 (2001): 242–73.

Beechy, Debra. "How Facial Hair Influences Women's Everyday Experiences," Master's thesis, Center for Humanistic Studies, Farmington, Michigan, 2004.

Benjamin, Harry. "Transsexualism and Transvestism as Psycho-Somatic and Somato-Psychic Syndromes," in *The Transgender Studies Reader*, ed. Susan Stryker and Stephen Whittle. New York: Routledge, 2006.

Benjamin, Jessica. *The Bonds of Love.* New York: Pantheon, 1988.

Bjorklund, David, and Pellegrini, Anthony. "Child Development and Evolutionary Psychology," *Child Development* 71 (2000): 1687–1708.

Borges, Jorge Luis. "The Analytical Language of John Wilkins," *Other Inquisitions, 1937–1952*, trans. Ruth Simms. Austin: University of Texas Press, 1964.

Bowman, Cameron, and Goldberg, Joshua. *Care of the Patient Undergoing Sex Reassignment Surgery*, Vancouver Coastal Health, 2006.

Brettell, Caroline, and Sargent, Carolyn (eds). *Gender in Cross-Cultural Perspective.* Englewood Cliffs, NJ: Prentice Hall, 1993.

Brody, Leslie. "The Socialization of Gender Differences in Emotional Expression: Display Rules, Infant Temperament, and Differentiation," in *Gender and Emotion: Social Psychological Perspectives*, ed. Agneta Fischer. Cambridge: Cambridge University Press, 2000.

Buller, David. "Evolutionary Psychology: The Emperor's New Paradigm," *TRENDS in Cognitive Sciences* 9 (2005): 277–83.

Butler, Judith. *Gender Trouble: Feminism and the Subversion of Identity.* New York: Routledge Classics, 2006.

Cahill, Larry. "Why Sex Matters for Neuroscience," *Nature Reviews: Neuroscience* 7 (2006): 477–84.

Catton, Chris, and James Gray. *Sex in Nature*. London: Croom Helm, 1985.

Chase, Cheryl. "Hermaphrodites with Attitude: Mapping the Emergence of Intersex Political Activism," in *The Transgender Studies Reader*, ed. Susan Stryker and Stephen Whittle. New York: Routledge, 2006.

Chivers, Meredith et al. "A Sex Difference in the Specificity of Sexual Arousal," *Psychological Science* 15 (2004): 736–44.

Coen, Enrico. *The Art of Genes: How Organisms Make Themselves*. Oxford: Oxford University Press, 1999.

Colapinto, John. "Gender Gap: What were the Real Reasons behind David Reimer's Suicide?" *Slate*, 3 June 2004.

Couch, Murray et al. *TranZnation: A Report on the Health and Wellbeing of Transgender People in Australia and New Zealand*, Melbourne: Australian Research Centre in Sex, Health and Society, 2007.

Dawkins, Richard. *The Ancestor's Tale*, Phoenix and London: Houghton Mifflin, 2005.

———. *The Blind Watchmaker*. London: Penguin, 2006.

Deary, Ian et al. "The Neuroscience of Human Intelligence Differences," *Nature Reviews: Neuroscience* 11 (2010): 201–11.

Diamond, Jared. "Father's Milk," *Discover*, February 1995.

Diamond, Milton, and Sigmundson, H. Keith. "Sex Reassignment at Birth," *The Nature-Nurture Debate: The Essential Readings*. Oxford: Blackwell, 1999.

Doidge, Norman. *The Brain that Changes Itself*. Melbourne: Scribe, 2007.

Drake, Emma. *What a Young Wife Ought to Know*. Philadelphia: The Vir Publishing Company, 1908.

Dreger, Alice Domurat. *Hermaphrodites and the Medical Invention of Sex*. Cambridge, MA: Harvard University Press, 1998.

Drews, Ulrich. *Color Atlas of Embryology*. New York: Thieme, 1995.

England, Paula et al. "Hooking Up and Forming Romantic Relationships on Today's College Campuses," in *The Gendered Society Reader*, ed. Michael Kimmel and Amy Aronson. Oxford: Oxford University Press, 2011.

Erikson, Erik. *Identity: Youth and Crisis*. London: Faber & Faber, 1968.

Eshagian, Tannaz (director). *Transsexual in Iran*. 2008.

Estioko-Griffin, Agnes, and Griffin, P. Bion. "Woman the Hunter: The Agta," *Gender in Cross-Cultural Perspective*, ed. Caroline Brettell and Carolyn Sargent. Englewood Cliffs, NJ: Prentice Hall, 1993.

Eugenides, Jeffrey. *Middlesex*. London: Bloomsbury, 2002.

European Association of Urology & European Society for Paediatric Urology. *Guidelines on Paediatric Urology*. Arnhem, 2009.

Family Court of Australia. "Re Alex: Hormonal Treatment for Gender Identity Dysphoria," 2004, FamCA 297.

———. "Re Brodie' (Special Medical Procedure), 2008, FamCA 334.

Fausto-Sterling, Anne. *Myths of Gender: Biological Theories about Women and Men*. New York: Basic Books, 1985.

———. *Sexing the Body: Gender Politics and the Construction of Sexuality*. New York: Basic Books, 2000.

———. "The Five Sexes: Why Male and Female are not Enough," *The Sciences* (March/April 1993): 20–24.

———. "The Five Sexes, Revisited," *The Sciences* 40 (July/August 2000): 18–23.

Feingold, Alan. "Cognitive Gender Differences are Disappearing," *American Psychologist* 43 (1988): 95–103.

Fisher, Ronald. *The Genetical Theory of Natural Selection*. Oxford: Oxford University Press, 1999.

Food and Agriculture Organization of the United Nations. "Women and Rural Employment: Fighting Poverty by Redefining Gender Roles," *Economic and Social Perspectives: Policy Brief 5* (August 2009).

Foucault, Michel. *The Order of Things: An Archaeology of the Human Sciences*. London: Tavistock Publications, 1970.

Fujimura, Joan. "Sex Genes: A Critical Sociomaterial Approach to the Politics and Molecular Genetics of Sex Determination," *Signs: Journal of Women in Culture and Society* 32 (2006): 49–82.

Garamszegi, Lázló, and Møller, Anders. "Extrapair Paternity and the Evolution of Bird Song," *Behavioral Ecology* 15 (2004): 508–19.

Garrod, Batten, and Thursfield, *Diseases of Children*, 4th ed. London: Edward Arnold & Co, 1947.

Georgiadis, Janniko et al. "Regional Cerebral Blood Flow Changes Associated with Clitorally Induced Orgasm in Healthy Women," *European Journal of Neuroscience* 24 (2006): 3305–16.

Gettler, Lee T. et al. "Longitudinal Evidence that Fatherhood Decreases Testosterone in Human Males," *Proceedings of the National Academy of Sciences* 2011; 108: 16194–9.

Gilmore, David. "The Manhood Puzzle," *Gender in Cross-Cultural Perspective*, ed. Caroline Brettell and Carolyn Sargent. Englewood Cliffs, NJ: Prentice Hall, 1993.

Graves, Jennifer. "Human Y Chromosome, Sex Differentiation, and Spermatogenesis—A Feminist View," *Biology of Reproduction* 63 (2000): 667–76.

———. "Sex Chromosome Specialization and Degeneration in Mammals," *Cell* 124 (2006): 901–14.

———. "The Rise and Fall of *SRY*," *TRENDS in Genetics* 18 (2002): 259–64.

Gray, John. *Men are from Mars, Women are from Venus: A Practical Guide for Improving Communication and Getting What You Want in Your Relationships*. London: Thorsons, 1993.

Haier, Richard et al. "The Neuroanatomy of General Intelligence: Sex Matters," *NeuroImage* 25 (2005): 320–27.

Harcourt, Christine et al. "The Health and Welfare Needs of Female and Transgender Street Sex Workers in New South Wales," *Australian and New Zealand Journal of Public Health* 25 (2007): 84–89.

Hare, Lauren et al. "Androgen Receptor Repeat Length Polymorphism Associated with Male-to-Female Transsexualism," *Biological Psychiatry* 65 (2009): 93–96.

Head, Jonathan. "Thai School Offers Transsexual Toilet," *BBC News*, 29 July 2008.

Henderson, Mark. "Women Fall into 'Trance' during Orgasm," *Times Online*, 20 June 2005.

Herdt, Gilbert. *Same Sex, Different Cultures: Exploring Gay and Lesbian Lives*. Boulder, CO: Westview Press, 1997.

Hitsch, Guenther et al. "What Makes You Click? Mate Preferences and Matching Outcomes in Online Dating," MIT Sloan School of Management, Research Paper No. 4603–6, February 2006.

Hoeft, Fumiko et al. "Gender Differences in the Mesocorticolimbic System during Computer Game-Play," *Journal of Psychiatric Research* 42 (2008): 253–58.

Holstege, Gert et al. "Brain Activation during Human Male Ejaculation," *The Journal of Neuroscience* 23 (2003): 9185–93.

Hunter, R. H. F. *Sex Determination, Differentiation and Intersexuality in Placental Mammals*. Cambridge: Cambridge University Press, 1995.

Huxlin, Krystel et al. "Perceptual Relearning of Complex Visual Motion after V1 Damage in Humans," *The Journal of Neuroscience* 29 (2009): 3981–91.

Hyde, Janet Shibley. "The Gender Similarities Hypothesis," *American Psychologist* 60 (2005): 581–92.

The Independent, "The Breasts a Man Can Get: Why 'Moobs' are no Laughing Matter," 7 March 2009 [no byline].

International Association of Athletics Federations. *IAAF Medical Manual*, "Chapter 13: Special Issues of Female Athletes," undated, www.iaaf.org/mm.

Jackson, Peter. "An Explosion of Thai Identities: Global Queering and Reimagining of Queer Theory," *Culture, Health and Sexuality* 2 (2000): 405–24.

———. "Tolerant but Unaccepting: The Myth of a Thai Gay Paradise," *Genders and Sexualities in Modern Thailand*, ed. Peter Jackson and Nerida Cook. Chiang Mai: Silkworm Books, 1999.

Jenkins, Rebecca. "Reasons for Surge in Hypospadias Remain Unclear," *Australian Doctor*, 12 April 2007.

Johannesen-Schmidt, Mary, and Eagly, Alice. "Another Look at Sex Differences in Preferred Mate Characteristics: The Effects of Endorsing the Traditional Female Gender Role," *Psychology of Women Quarterly* 26 (2002): 322–28.

Jones, James Holland. *Monkey's Uncle* blog, http://monkeysuncle.stanford.edu/.

Jones, Richard. *Human Reproductive Biology*. San Diego: Academic Press, 1997.

Jones, Steve. *Y: The Descent of Men*. London: Abacus, 2002.

Kessler, Suzanne, and McKenna, Wendy. "Toward a Theory of Gender," in *The Transgender Studies Reader*, ed. Susan Stryker and Stephen Whittle. New York: Routledge, 2006.

Kimmel, Michael, and Aronson, Amy. *The Gendered Society Reader*. New York: Oxford University Press, 2011.

Komisaruk, Barry et al. *The Science of Orgasm*. Baltimore: The Johns Hopkins University Press, 2006.

Koopman, Peter et al. "Male Development of Chromosomally Female Mice Transgenic for *Sry*," *Nature* 351 (1991): 117–21.

Kramer, Heinrich, and Sprenger, James. *The Malleus Maleficarum*, trans. Montague Summers. Mineola, NY: Dover Publications, 1971.

Lamphere, Louise. "The Domestic Sphere of Women and the Public World of Men: The Strengths and Limitations of an Anthropological Dichotomy," *Gender in Cross-Cultural Perspective*, ed. Caroline Brettell and Carolyn Sargent. Englewood Cliffs, NJ: Prentice Hall, 1993.

Larsen, William J. *Essentials of Human Embryology*, Churchill Livingstone, 1998.

Leaper, Campbell, and Friedman, Carly Kay. "The Socialization of Gender," *Handbook of Socialization: Theory and Research*, ed. Joan Grusec and Paul Hastings. New York: Guilford Publications, 2007.

LeBon, Gustave. "Recherches anatomiques et mathematiques sur les lois des variations du volume du cerveau et sur leurs relations avec l'intelligence," *Revue d'Anthropologie* 2 (1879): 27–104 (my translation).

Levy, Ariel. "Either/Or: Sports, Sex and the Case of Caster Semenya," *The New Yorker*, November 2009.

Maccoby, Eleanor. *The Two Sexes: Growing up Apart, Coming Together*. Cambridge, MA: Harvard University Press, 1998.

Morgan, Elaine. *The Descent of Women*. New York: Bantam Books, 1977.

Nanda, Serena. "Hijras as neither Man nor Woman," in *The Lesbian and Gay Studies Reader*, ed. Henry Abelove et al. New York: Routledge, 1993.

———. "The *Hijras* of India: Cultural and Individual Dimensions of an Institutionalized Third Gender Role," in *Culture, Society and Sexuality: A Reader*, 2nd ed., ed. Richard Parker and Peter Aggleton. London and New York: Routledge, 2003.

Nsubuga, Anthony et al. "Patterns of Paternity and Group Fission in Wild Multimale Mountain Gorilla Groups," *American Journal of Physical Anthropology* 135 (2008): 263–74.

Parafianowicz, Lydia. "Swedish Parents Keep Two-Year-Old's Gender Secret," *The Local: Sweden's News in English*, 23.6.09, www.thelocal.se/20232/20090623/.

Penton-Voak, I. S. et al. "Menstrual Cycle Alters Face Preference," *Nature* 399 (1999): 741–42.

Peplau, Letitia. "Human Sexuality: How do Men and Women Differ?" *Current Directions in Psychological Science* 12 (2003): 37–40.

Perrett, D. I. et al. "Effects of Sexual Dimorphism on Facial Attractiveness," *Nature* 394 (1998): 84–87.

Pinker, Steven. *The Blank Slate: The Modern Denial of Human Nature*. New York: Penguin, 2002.

Preves, Sharon. *Intersex and Identity: The Contested Self*. New Brunswick, NJ: Rutgers University Press, 2005.

Raymond, Janice. "Sappho by Surgery: The Transsexually Constructed Lesbian Feminist," in *The Transgender Studies Reader*, ed. Susan Stryker and Stephen Whittle. New York: Routledge, 2006.

Reay, Diane. "'Spice Girls,' 'Nice Girls,' 'Girlies,' and 'Tomboys': Gender Discourses, Girls' Cultures, and Femininities in the Primary Classroom," *The Gendered Society Reader*, ed. Michael Kimmel and Amy Aronson. Oxford: Oxford University Press, 2011 [sic].

Reeser, J. C. "Gender Identity and Sport: Is the Playing Field Level?" *British Journal of Sports Medicine* 39 (2005): 695–99.

Reichard, Ulrich. "Extra-pair Copulations in a Monogamous Gibbon," *Ethology* 100 (1995): 99–112.

Ridley, Matt. *Nature via Nurture: Genes, Experience and What Makes Us Human*. London: Harper Perennial, 2004.

———. *The Origins of Virtue*. London: Penguin, 1997.

Roach, Mary. *Bonk: The Curious Coupling of Science and Sex*. New York: W. W. Norton & Co., 2008.

Rogers, Lesley. "Extreme Problems with Essential Differences," *Cerebrum* 5 (2003): 88–95.

———. *Sexing the Brain*. London: Weidenfeld & Nicolson, 1999.

Rood, Kate. "The Sea Horse, Our Family Mascot," *New York Times*, 2 November 2008.

Rosin, Hanna. "A Boy's Life," *The Atlantic Monthly*, November 2008.

Ruble, Diane, and Martin, Carol. "Gender Development," *Handbook of Child Psychology, Volume 3: Social, Emotional and Personal Development*, ed. Nancy Eisenberg. Hoboken, NJ: John Wiley & Sons, 1996.

Scherer, G., and M. Schmid (eds). *Genes and Mechanisms in Vertebrate Sex Determination*. Basel: Birkhaueser, 2001.

Schmitt, David. "Sociosexuality from Argentina to Zimbabwe: A 48-nation study of sex, culture, and strategies of human mating," *Behavioural and Brain Sciences* 28 (2005): 247–311.

Short, Robert (chaired). *The Genetics and Biology of Sex Determination*. Chichester, UK: John Wiley & Sons, 2002.

Sjöström, Mia. "Pojke eller flicker? Det säger vi inte," *Svenska Dagbladet*, 6 March 2009 (translated with the assistance of Anna McCredie).

Spade, Dean. "Mutilating Gender," in *The Transgender Studies Reader*, ed. Susan Stryker and Stephen Whittle. New York: Routledge, 2006.

Stanford, Craig. "The Social Behavior of Chimpanzees and Bonobos: Empirical Evidence and Shifting Assumptions," *Current Anthropology* 39 (1998): 399–420 (includes responses).

Stoller, Robert. *Sex and Gender: The Development of Masculinity and Femininity*. Oxford: Science House, 1968.

Stopes, Marie. *Married Love: A New Contribution to the Solution of Sex Difficulties*, 21st ed. London: Putnam & Co., 1934 (first published 1918).

Stryker, Susan, and Whittle, Stephen. *The Transgender Studies Reader*. New York: Routledge, 2006.

Tannen, Deborah. *You Just Don't Understand: Women and Men in Conversation*. London: Random House, 1990.

Thorne, Barrie. "Children and Gender: Constructions of Difference," in *Toward a New Psychology of Gender: A Reader*, ed. Mary Gergen and Sara Davis. New York: Routledge, 1997.

Trut, Lyudmila. "Early Canid Domestication: The Farm Fox Experiment," *American Scientist* 87 (1999): 160–69.

Udry, J. Richard. "Biological Limits of Gender Construction," *American Sociological Review* 65 (2000): 443–57.

Van der Meer, Theo. "Eugenic and Sexual Folklores and the Castration of Sex Offenders in the Netherlands (1938–1968)," *Studies in History and Philosophy of Biological and Biomedical Sciences* 39 (2008); 195–204.

Vilain, Eric. "Anomalies of Human Sexual Development: Clinical Aspects and Genetic Analysis," in *The Genetics and Biology of Sex Determination*, chaired by Robert Short. Chichester, UK: John Wiley & Sons, 2002.

Voight, Benjamin et al. "A Map of Recent Positive Selection in the Human Genome," *PloS Biology* 4 (2006): e72.

Warne, Garry et al. "A Long-term Outcome Study of Intersex Conditions," *Journal of Pediatric Endocrinology & Metabolism* 18 (2005): 555–67.

West, Candace, and Zimmerman, Don. "Doing Gender," *The Gendered Society Reader*, ed. Michael Kimmel and Amy Aronson, Oxford University Press, Oxford, 2011 [sic].

Wharton, Amy. *The Sociology of Gender: An Introduction to Theory and Research*. Oxford: Blackwell, 2005.

Wilhelm, Dagmar, and Koopman, Peter. "The Makings of Maleness: Towards an Integrated View of Male Sexual Development," *Nature* 7 (August 2006).

Wilhelm, Dagmar et al. "Sex Determination and Gonadal Development in Mammals," *Physiological Reviews* 87 (2007): 1–28.

Williams, Walter. "Amazons of America: Female Gender Variance," *Gender in Cross-Cultural Perspective*, ed. Caroline Brettell and Carolyn Sargent. Englewood Cliffs, NJ: Prentice Hall, 1993.

Winston, Robert. *The Human Mind*, Bantam Books, London, 2003.

Index

.

About the Author

Jane McCredie is an award-winning Sydney-based journalist, writer, and editor. The former news and features editor at Australia's leading weekly magazine for doctors, she has a longstanding interest in psychology and holds a Master of Arts in psychosocial studies from the University of Melbourne.